An Excellent Choice

An
Excellent
Choice

===

PANIC AND JOY

ON MY SOLO PATH

TO MOTHERHOOD

===

Emma Brockes

PENGUIN PRESS

NEW YORK » 2018

PENGUIN PRESS
An imprint of Penguin Random House LLC
375 Hudson Street
New York, New York 10014
penguin.com

LIBRARY OF CONGRESS CATALOGING-IN-PUBLICATION DATA

Names: Brockes, Emma, author.
Title: An excellent choice: panic and joy on my solo path to motherhood /
    Emma Brockes.
Description: New York: Penguin Press, 2018.
Identifiers: LCCN 2018006198 (print) | LCCN 2018009187 (ebook) |
    ISBN 9780698402621 (ebook) | ISBN 9781594206634 (hardcover)
Subjects: LCSH: Brockes, Emma—Health. | Fertilization in vitro,
    Human—Biography. | Infertility, Female—Patients—England—
    Biography. |
    Mothers—England—Biography. | BISAC: BIOGRAPHY &
    AUTOBIOGRAPHY / Personal
    Memoirs. | HEALTH & FITNESS / Pregnancy & Childbirth. | HUMOR /
    Topic / Marriage & Family.
Classification: LCC RG135 (ebook) | LCC RG135 .B74 2018 (print) | DDC
    618.1/780599092 [B] —dc23
LC record available at https://lccn.loc.gov/2018006198

Printed in the United States of America
10 9 8 7 6 5 4 3 2 1

Designed by Marysarah Quinn

The names and identifying characteristics of certain individuals
have been changed to protect their privacy.

For my family

Contents

An Excellent Choice

Prologue

EIGHT P.M. IS A DANGEROUS TIME in my household. If everything has gone well in the preceding few hours, two out of the three of us will be sleeping, but it's a light sleep, easily broken. If everything has gone badly, two will be wailing. There is an indeterminate stage, when one is asleep and one wakes up, in which case I have approximately four and a half seconds from the sound of the first murmur to rise from the sofa, skid down the hall in my socks, cross the bedroom in two Spiderman-style leaps and soothe her to sleep before she yells and wakes up the other one. This is what it is to be outnumbered by one's children: you are always ready to run.

The anxiety of bedtime is known to all parents—the fact that for babies under two, the trajectory from afternoon into evening must be negotiated with the precision of a space shuttle reentering the earth's atmosphere (too steep and you will trigger the baby's indignant rage; too shallow and she will bounce off into overtiredness, never to return)—but it is felt most acutely, perhaps, by single parents. For us, the danger of evening isn't only in the wailing, the stress and the tiredness. It is in those close-of-day hours when we are inclined to feel the strangeness of our circumstance most keenly—in my case, the manifold strangeness of being a Briton in Manhattan and a single mother of twin girls, with a partner, or partner-of-sorts, who lives with her three-year-old son in the apartment upstairs.

This scenario is not the fruit of careful planning. Even five years ago, when I first started thinking that if I wanted a baby then I'd better get on with it, all my imagination would stretch to was the blurry outline of a small, portable infant whom I could pop into my bag and take with me on jobs to L.A., or out to dinner in New York, where it would lie quietly in its car seat under the table. It would have my surname and dark hair like me, and if it was a boy, I'd raise him gay so we could watch old musicals together on Sunday afternoons. If it was a girl, she'd be bookish and serious with straight bangs across her forehead, like a smaller version of Amelie, or Matilda without the telekinesis.

How this baby would come into being I had no idea, but given that I was, at the time, living alone in a walk-up in Brooklyn, with unstable immigration status and a fluctuating income, I had a few things to figure out first. I was also in a relationship with a woman. L was three years older than me and wanted a baby, too, which would seem to offer an obvious route toward a somewhat conventional family arrangement. The only problem was this: we didn't want the same baby.

Before I go on, I should say that L is not a writer and finds the endless use to which I put my own life distasteful—I can't imagine why—and so, in the story that follows, the ins and outs of our relationship aren't something I can get overly into. What I can say is this: she and I were not twenty-two-year-old newlyweds. We were women in our late thirties who, when we met, had been around long enough to know our own natures and be somewhat unflinching in regard to accommodating them. She did not want a baby as an expression of her love for me. I did not want a baby as a reflection of my love for her. I wanted a baby because I wanted a baby, and if I'm forced to give more of a reason than that, the best I can do is to say that, as in most things, from how I make scrambled eggs (with water, not milk) to how I fight (indirectly), concede (grudgingly), compete (overly), love (jealously) and hate (over decades, and with an overdeveloped appetite for revenge), it probably has to do with the relationship I had with my mother. Anyway, whatever it was, it had nothing to do with the person I was seeing.

Clearly this presented me with a number of problems. The choices available to thirty-six-year-old single women who want babies have not, historically, been wildly attractive. You can get lucky. You can get promiscuous. You can, as women essayists pop up every few years to remind us, "settle" for a partner you're not wholly into, that is, if you can find someone abject enough to agree. You can turn your life upside down at the first whiff of romance. In the past few years, I have watched as friends, or friends of friends, have moved from New York to St. Louis, the West Coast, London or, in the most extreme case, Bali to be with a man. ("I win!" said the one who went to Bali.) These women, all aware of and grimly amused by this trend, put it this way: you can live in New York and never meet anyone or you can move to the other side of the world, change your job, abandon your friends, but win the jackpot of being in a couple. (The landscape is slightly different for single gay friends, who have better luck in the cities, but suffer the same uncertainty as to whether the person they've met is the "right" one to have kids with.) No man I know has, in the early stages of a relationship, ever moved to where his girlfriend was living unless he had at least one other good reason for doing so.

There are two further possibilities: resign yourself to the fact it's not going to happen, or pull the emergency cord and do it alone.

I should pause here to acknowledge that being a single parent is still, for the most part, not a matter of choice but of unforeseen circumstance and as such makes what I'm talking about—elective single motherhood—laughably decadent, a bunch of well-heeled professional women fretting over how to have babies, when the vast majority of single mothers are just trying to get by. Of the ten million single parents in the United States, eight million of whom are women, nearly half live below the poverty line.

The very definition of single parenthood exists on a sliding scale, and because competition over who has it worst is often as fierce as it is over who has it best, I should also own to the fact that having L upstairs insulates me from many of the anxieties of raising babies alone. Single mothers with no help at all will feel superior to me, just as I feel superior to divorcées with big alimony settlements or anyone with fewer than two babies or women who have their own mothers on hand, and we all feel superior to married women who say things like "Dave's off golfing and I'm a single mum for the weekend!"

This petty machismo is, in my experience, outmeasured by the solidarity among women raising kids on their own, but in any case, this is not a book about my life as a single parent, the difficulties of which are comparatively small and ordinary compared with those of the period immediately preceding it. These were the months and years of my mid- to late thirties when every day seemed to bring another set of terrifying and uniquely irreversible decisions. Am I really going to do this? How am I going to do this? How much will it cost? Can I afford it? How alone will I be? Where will we live? Is it too weird? What if my kid doesn't look like me? Is it immoral? What if it doesn't work? What if it does work? Can I use it as an anchor baby? Am I ready to be a single mother? How I negotiated these decisions in the midst of all the advice, scolding and general hysteria that still attends the way in which a woman has, or doesn't have, children is the main concern of this book.

I will not be writing about elective single dads, not out of any bias against them but because I know so few—one, in fact. It is, however, fair to assume that aside from the stuff about vaginas and ovaries, most of what I'm saying here applies equally to them. In fact, because of assumptions about men's nurturing abilities and the narrower range of biological options available to them, men wanting children alone probably have it harder than we do.

Still, the vast majority of people choosing to become single parents at the moment are women. As I write, two of my oldest friends are pregnant with babies conceived the same way that mine were, two others are trying and it's no exaggeration to say that, of those who want children, every other single or kind-of-single woman I know is considering it. "It's the death of men," said a (married) friend recently, a little caustically, I thought. "No," I said. "It's the death of crappy relationships for the sake of having a baby." It's the death of back-against-the-wall decision making. It is, potentially, the death of a lot of unhappiness, although ask me again in thirty years' time when my own children's memoirs come out. In any case, it is the rise of options where latterly there were none.

What it isn't, I'm pretty sure, is the THIN END OF THE WEDGE, the slippery slope into eugenics and a master race and curated children with no sense of belonging. In Denmark, where they have, of course, been doing it for years, one in ten babies conceived with donor sperm is born to a single mother by choice and nascent studies show that the kids are all right, performing across every metric as well as or above children from traditional two-parent families. Even so, the notion of a sperm donor, while more socially acceptable than that of an egg donor or a surrogate, comes with hefty negative connotations. It is selfish. It is existentially troubling. It messes up the children. It messes up society. It encourages women to leave it later and later to have a first child, with the concurrent risks to both mother and baby. Since my babies were born, I have been informed by one news outlet or another that they pose a threat to democracy, god's good grace, evolutionary design, the sanctity of marriage, human diversity, common decency, male self-esteem and themselves. Not bad for two people who can't say their own names yet.

To them, then, I offer this scene, a fade-out from the bookish, dark-haired baby of my dreams to two flame-haired toddlers in a Taco Bell off I-495. We have stopped for dinner on the way out to Long Island, where we are vacationing for a week with L and her son. She is holding two children, one hers, one mine, both grabbing at her car keys while she tries to order three Meximelts and a chicken burrito. My other daughter is squirming in my arms, pointing to people in the restaurant and, in an accent none of us knows how she came by but that has for the past few months made me feel as if I were living with a small, angry German woman, shouting her signature phrase, "Oh no! Vhat's THAT?"

For a week we will sleep, eat and play together on the beach, and when we return from vacation, we will ride up in the elevator together until my children and I get out on the seventeenth floor and L and hers proceed to the eighteenth. As I do every night, I will put them to bed alone, hovering outside the door like a criminal to ensure they've gone down before eating dinner in front of the TV and doing the 101 things that go into maintaining two toddlers. I will rinse the bottles and put them in the dishwasher. I will tidy the toys and grill chicken for the girls' lunch the next day. I will worry about the rash behind the smaller girl's knees and why the bigger one isn't walking yet. Before I go to bed, I will look in the fridge, curse myself for forgetting to buy milk and wonder whether, come the morning, I will be noble enough to give what's left to my children or, in the manner of fix-your-own-mask-before-helping-others, use the last dregs in my coffee. At ten p.m., I will go to bed alone and by the morning there will be three of us in the bed, our breath rising and falling in unison.

That none of this makes sense doesn't diminish its power to amaze me, not because of how I got here, although god knows there were enough ups, downs and pharmaceuticals along the way. Instead, what I wonder at in the off hours is how a contingency plan, a so-called measure of last resort that I was supposed to hope against hope wouldn't be my fate, somehow became my first and best choice.

ONE

"Are You Going to Do It, Then?"

THE HARDEST THING about having a baby alone isn't the expense, the fear or the loneliness. It isn't the process of getting pregnant, with its cycles of raised and dashed hopes, or the term "sperm donor," with its unsettling connotations. It's not even the queasy feeling, indistinct but pervasive, that what you are doing sets you apart from other people and that the reason you are doing it is not because you are a powerful, rational, resourceful woman, but, as a friend of mine put it recently after considering and rejecting the idea of having a baby alone, because "I couldn't get anyone to shag me."

All of these things are hard, but they are not the hardest. No. The hardest thing about having a baby alone is making the decision to do it.

"So are you going to do it, then?" says Rosemary. It is late in the summer of 2013 and we are drinking whiskey in a hotel bar in Edinburgh. Rosemary is in the city to attend a panel at the Edinburgh Book

Festival, where I am promoting a book. I have spent the afternoon in a deck chair on the festival lawn, watching literary men with large hair sail by and trying to figure out a strategy for getting up.

"Yeah, probably," I say. "I mean, I might do. Are you?"

"I don't know."

I haven't seen Rosemary for a few months and we have a lot to catch up on: her new job, my new book, the fortunes of all the people we both know. It is only after more whiskey, however, and with a casualness that belies the cold, flat terror underneath, that we reach the main order of business: our ongoing discussion, part lament, part spur to action, over what to do about having children. That is: if, when, how and with whom, or rather, since we are both, for the purposes of this conversation, single, "with" "whom." (Neither of us yet knows this, but there are more air quotes in the world of assisted fertility than there are in a vegan cookbook.)

"The thing is," says Rosemary, "what if it turns out fugly?"

"You get pictures of the donor. Also, I thought you said your friend was obese." The last time I saw Rosemary, she told me she'd been thinking of using her best friend, a larger gentleman, as a sperm donor, since when he'd got a new girlfriend and nixed it.

"He is," she says. "It's different when you know him, though."

I have always known I wanted children. From the time I was old enough to conceptualize my future, motherhood made sense to me, the way books made sense to me and equations did not. It was always one in my imaginings and never part of a fantasy about marriage, and while everything else in my life changed over the years—the country I lived in, the kind of work I did, the gender of the people I dated—the distant outline of a child remained steadfast. For a long time it was in the deep background, a passive assumption rather an active desire, and yet on the rare occasions I allowed myself to inspect it directly, the idea that it might never happen made me feel giddy with loss.

There is deciding you want a baby in the far distant future, however, and there is deciding to have one right now, alone, and those two things are wholly distinct. I should say at this point that despite surface indicators to the contrary, I am pretty conventional. I began paying into a pension fund at twenty-three. I bought my first property at twenty-five. I didn't start moisturizing until too late, but in most other respects, I spent the bulk of my twenties conscientiously working my way through the world's most sensible to-do list. Before the question of babies came up, the most radical thing I'd ever done was to resign from my job of eight years and move from Britain to America, a less risky move than it sounds given that on the day after my resignation, I signed a short-term contract to do the same job for the same company but on slightly worse terms.

I was thirty-one years old and America was, if not the shining city on a hill, then the promise of every eighties movie I had ever seen. When people asked why I had moved, the flippant answer I gave was that it was a result of coming of age in the era of *Working Girl* and *Desperately Seeking Susan*. There was probably some truth to this. It was almost impossible to grow up in Britain in the 1980s and not see New York as a city of outlandish good fortune, a place where people dried their armpits under the hand dryers in the Greyhound bus station toilets or took the Staten Island Ferry to work, walking in as the secretary and out again as CEO. Where we had Kim Wilde, they had Madonna. Where we had the BT Tower, they had the Empire State Building. They had hustle, we had wait-your-turn and be-grateful-for-what-you-get. And while the New York media was, I was sure, the red beating heart of the entire universe, by the time I left London, its British equivalent had started to feel like a fish tank that didn't get cleaned out enough.

I wasn't thinking about babies when I got to New York. I was thinking how liberating it was to be far from home. It was the run up to the 2008 presidential election and I spent a lot of that first winter standing in frozen parking lots in Iowa, trying to understand the difference between a caucus and a primary. Simple things became strange. No one knew what I meant when I said "sockets" or "loo paper" and when I judged something to be "quite good," most Americans thought I meant it was quite good, rather than what I obviously meant, which is that it was terrible. Even lunch in America was exciting. It is hard to remain jaded about life when embedded in the mere act of ordering a sandwich is the drama of having to say "tomato" three times.

And while I was friendless in those first weeks and months, wandering around Central Park at the weekend with a twenty-dollar salad from Whole Foods and no one to talk to, this too, in its way, was quite thrilling. You can be bolder when there's an ocean between you and everyone you know, something that mostly manifests in small acts of transgression, like ordering takeout every night or bunking off to drink champagne on a weekday or pretending to be the sort of person who can carry off leopard print, but that one day, I hoped, might give me the push to make more radical life choices. In the meantime, I could write off months, and even years, futzing around trying to figure out where to live, or how to get a Social Security number, or where to buy cheese that didn't taste of emulsified plastic.

The real reason I had moved to America—the one I was willing to admit to—was to buy myself time to write a book about my mother, and any thought of babies, along with everything else in my life, fell effortlessly into the category of Things I Can't Possibly Do Until I've Finished The Book. Every day, I sat in the small second bedroom I used as an office surrounded by bits of paper and photos, books stacked haphazardly on the floor, a plant in a green vase with a crack across it in the window, and tried to put my mother's life into words. I went for long walks around my East Village neighborhood, deliberating over who she had been. The easy part was that I was her only child and the love of her life and that she was my great champion and friend. She played Scrabble with me on rainy afternoons and took me to the jewelry store where she worked, where I played on the adding machine and counted the money. She sat with me through old musicals and made me read *Gone with the Wind*. She filled me with a sense of my own consequence and the idea that my best was always enough. "Have the courage of your insane convictions," she said. And, "Of course you can do it, you're my child." And, "If at first you don't succeed . . ."

This was my mother as I knew her when I was a child. But there was another story, much of which I found out about only after her death from lung cancer in 2003. If, as adults, we are engaged in continuous acts of trying either to replicate our childhoods or to get as far away from them as possible, then my mother fell into the latter category. She had left South Africa for England in 1960 ostensibly for political reasons but for what turned out to be personal ones. Adults who have been abused as children bring a very particular set of assumptions to the raising of their own children, and the fierceness of my mother's love for me, and the ways in which it came out, were rooted in what turned out to be the extraordinary traumas of her childhood. It shouldn't be surprising that she, a motherless child whose father was a violent alcoholic and pedophile, should have married my dad, a kind, loving, generous man with whom she could make a safe home for herself and their child, nor that she should choose to live in a part of the world—a leafy village in the south of England—where the worst thing that would ever happen to her was living next door to someone who had voted for Thatcher.

It was a conventional household: my dad, a lawyer, made the money; my mum, a part-time bookkeeper, kept the home. But she was not a conventional woman. She had the very un-English habit of talking to people in shops and queues. She was confrontational, the kind of mother who told off other people's children in the dentist's waiting room while I slouched down in my seat for shame. I took it for granted that, compared with other people's mothers, my mother was just More: bigger, louder, stronger and of course she loved me more than their mothers loved them, not through any fault of theirs, but as a simple matter of physics. My mother had survived unimaginable abuse as a child and, as a result, had a sense not only of life's fragility but of its possibility, too, of how far one might travel from any given point of origin, evidence for which was the baby before her. "Those precious feet," she would say, taking me to the shoe shop for the umpteenth time for the woman to check whether I hadn't outgrown my shoes. "Those precious hands." "Those precious teeth."

Writing about these things, weighing up my mother's life and the impact of her mothering on me, dominated my first years in America, and as my midthirties loomed, what had started out as a joy turned into a nightmare; everything subordinated to getting the thing finished. Every few weeks, I broke off to make some money by writing a story for my newspaper and glance longingly toward the day when it would be over and I could finally tackle the rest of my to-do list: find a cheaper apartment, apply for a green card, tidy up, go to the dentist, find saucepans that worked for me, change my cable provider, do something about my hair, repot the plant, get more fiber in my diet, and confront this business of having or not having a baby.

That last consideration was one I pushed to the back every time. It was too big, too alarming, and a cliché to boot. Prioritizing children isn't what feminists *do,* I told myself, a corrective to millennia of their being a woman's only priority. Some of my friends had kids but most of them didn't, either because they didn't want them or because they didn't want them At All Costs. If there was regret and sadness that came with this, it was accompanied by the understanding that life entails choice and choice entails loss.

At least my life in New York had opened out by this time. When I met L, I was two thirds of the way toward finishing the book and ready to start going out again. On the surface of things, we looked very different—me, English, lefty, fundamentally unkempt; she, New Yorker, center right, well put together—although if one allows that British journalism and New York finance are two of the most aggressive industries in the world, then on some level we understood each other perfectly. "Everything is sales," she said one night not long after we met. We were in her apartment on the Upper East Side, where vague shouts drifted up from the Irish bar below. "That's a terrible way to look at the world," I said pompously and tried to figure out what I thought "everything" was. "Everything is story," I said eventually, and this seemed to me an insurmountable difference between us until I realized both entailed spending large amounts of time trying to recruit other people to one's own point of view. She was ferociously good at her job and I admired this, too.

Still, on any given day we could disagree about everything under the sun—fact or fiction, Manhattan or Brooklyn, subway or car, Republican or Democrat, all the way down to cats or dogs—so that in the months after we met, it felt like being on an extended safari in each other's alien worlds. I made her read Joan Didion and took her to press nights on Broadway. She made me read *Good to Great* and a memoir by Cathie Black, the former chairman of Hearst Magazines, and took me to a car dealership in Queens, where she bamboozled the salesman so thoroughly he practically paid her to take the car off the lot. If falling in love is, partly, a question of finding a docking station for one's neuroses, I knew I was home when L told me that after her building was evacuated during 9/11, she went straight to a liquor store and bought hundreds of dollars' worth of hard liquor in case civilization collapsed and the world reverted to a barter economy. Come the zombie apocalypse, this is a woman you want on your side. But there was this, too; the house she grew up in would one day have to be sold, she said, and what she would miss most were the things you can't take with you, like the sound the stairs made when they expanded at night. Somewhere in my system, a pilot light flared.

All relationships have a deadline by which they must either find their level or fall apart, but it is not as hard a deadline as the one on a woman's fertility, and, as she was three years older than me, L told me from the outset that in the near future, she was planning on trying to get pregnant. Logistically, this made sense; if she was sure she wanted a baby, it would be madness to forestall while we flapped about for another three years trying to decide what we were doing. Emotionally, however, it stumped me. According to every relationship model I knew, you could either be with someone who'd had kids before you met, have kids together and separate down the line or split up and have a baby alone. There was no such thing as being with someone who had a baby on her own, for the very good reason that it sounded like a terrible deal: all the stress and anxiety without the substance of motherhood, the rights and responsibilities that are the beginning of love.

At that stage, the strongest terms in which I could have put my own long-held but dormant desire for a baby were that I didn't want *not* to have one. Materially, I'm not terribly acquisitive. If I ever win the lottery,

I'll have to suppress a dickish urge to dash out and buy a Lamborghini, but in the ordinary run of things, I don't care much about bags or shoes or clothes or apartment size. What I am greedy for, like most writers and journalists, is insight, and on the rare occasions I gave it any thought, it drove me insane to consider the possibility that if I didn't have kids, any two-bit newlywed with a baby could lay claim to greater knowledge of human existence than I could. I thought of all the people I hated with children and grew faint with indignation and rage. If there was, behind this impulse, a larger, less tangible longing, I didn't want to look into it too deeply lest it unleash a full-blown baby hunger I couldn't get back in the box.

I did at least manage to move from Manhattan to a cheaper apartment in Brooklyn during those years, around the same time L moved apartments, so that for a very brief window we considered moving in together. After all, we had a lot of fun; we'd driven out to the beach for the summer and she'd come with me on a couple of jobs to L.A. We'd hired a convertible and driven from Las Vegas to Palm Springs, where we laughed ourselves silly playing hipster bingo at the Art Deco hotel. Without a financial incentive, however—I was low on funds, that far into writing a book, but I had low overheads, too, and was paid by my newspaper in sterling, still worth something then—moving in together wasn't appealing. I had too many books; she had too many clothes. I worked mainly from home and needed space for an office, which meant getting something bigger than either of us was willing to pay for. We also fought a lot. Our fights started out small and blew up to encompass everything. We fought in ways I had never fought with anyone, livid, shouting, crying (her), icy, cruel, withholding (me). "You have no needs," she once yelled, an insult that baffled me at the time. Surely having no needs was a form of perfection? (Thank you; the limitations of this position have since become clear to me.) After every argument, I thought, that's it, we're done, and the next day—truly one of the revelations of adulthood—we made up and moved on. Apparently conflict, which I try to avoid at all costs, can be managed as part of a healthy relationship.

It did, however, mean that the only way we could envisage living together was in a five-bedroom house arranged over three floors, so that in the event of a fight, we could retreat to different altitudes with an entire floor between us. Instead, we were looking at the standard New York two-bedroom, with barely enough space for one low-maintenance man, let alone two women. Things carried on as they were.

Or, they almost did. I started to notice small, unsettling changes in myself. When somebody asked me, "Do you have children?"—a question that, until recently, I had responded to in my head with versions of "Are you mental, I'm about eleven"—it started to sound less neutral, more unfriendly. At a friend's weeklong house party for her fortieth, I looked at the other guests, successful women all, most of whom were at least five years older than me and, with one exception, none of whom had children, and for the first time gave consideration to how they got there. I had always believed as a matter of principle that, medical issues aside, most women without children had acted through choice, but now my faith in this weakened. I watched as a number of friends missed out on having children because their boyfriends broke up with them when they were in the vicinity of forty, before going on to have children with younger women. I watched as women five, six, seven years my senior finally met someone new and went through round after punishing round of IVF. I let my mind drift back to a conversation I'd had with someone years earlier, an elderly friend of my mother's and a surrogate grandmother of sorts, whom I had loved and admired and who, as far as I knew, had been entirely content to have lived her life without children. Then visiting her one day around her ninetieth birthday, she clutched my hand out of the blue and, with an urgency that shocked me, said, "All that matters is children," a breach of character so startling I put it down to old age and sentiment, even though, after my mother, she was the least sentimental person I knew.

Slowly, I started to form visions of the future I didn't want to be mine. This is, I realize, inverse to the kind of advice doled out by books like *The Secret,* in which we are told that the key to getting what we want in life is to create a precise picture of it in our head and work slavishly and unwaveringly toward that one goal. Instead, looking back, I see that most of my decisions have been made by figuring out what I don't want, then doing everything in my power to make sure it doesn't happen. This may be because my dislikes are more violent than my appetites, but it also, it seems to me, allows for the possibility that there are more routes to happiness than we can imagine ahead of time.

I didn't want to be alone at forty-five in a walk-up in Brooklyn, or fifty and on Tinder, dating people with children when I had none of my own. I didn't want to be seventy, the age my mother was when she died, lying on my deathbed without the image of my child's face in my head. Above all, I didn't want to look back on this period, when there was still time to change things, and wish I'd had the courage to act.

I also didn't want to "help" another woman raise her baby. Unless I was Mother Teresa (I'm not), the only way it would make sense for me to stick around in the event of L's having a child was if our relationship changed to become a more conventional union, or—and this is where my imagination really started to strain at the leash—if I had my own baby independently, too.

. . .

THIS PERIOD OF PARALYSIS might have gone on indefinitely if, in the autumn of 2012, something strange hadn't happened. My youth, which in line with the rest of my generation had tapered obscenely on from my adolescence into my twenties and well into my thirties, came abruptly to an end. Ordinarily, I like odd-number birthdays; there's less pressure on them to be fun than on even numbers. I hadn't enjoyed my thirtieth much, but I'd liked turning twenty-nine and thirty-one. Thirty-three, when I had a joint party at a bar in downtown Manhattan that smelled exactly like London—of spilled beer and Windex—was a blast. That year, however, the run-up to my odd-numbered birthday was different. No matter how hard I looked at it, I couldn't convince myself that thirty-seven was still my midthirties. It was, indisputably, the start of my late thirties, which meant the next stop was forty, which meant that, according to every magazine article I had ever read on the subject, my reproductive system was about to knit itself a bed jacket and retire. It didn't matter that I wasn't broody. It didn't matter that I was in the wrong country, the wrong apartment, possibly—we hadn't decided yet—the wrong relationship. It didn't even matter if I wanted kids or not. What mattered was that if I didn't act now, or at least soon, the decision would be taken out of my hands.

I knew of a single example of a woman in her thirties having a baby alone through planning, not accident, and that was Tessa, my friend Laura's sister, who'd had two children via sperm donor a decade earlier. Tessa, an energetic and successful entrepreneur from the north of England, was someone I knew only slightly but whom I had for years admired from afar. She was a decade older than me and it was apparent from the way in which Laura talked about it that her decision to have two babies alone had been considered brave but somewhat scandalous. No one at her work knew how her kids were conceived, said Laura, and although it was all wonderful now, it had taken their dad in particular awhile to come round. I had shoved the example of Tessa to the back of my mind in a file marked Too Frightening To Think About Now But That Might One Day Turn Out To Be Useful and that's where it stayed, right up until that year I turned thirty-seven, which was also the year L got pregnant.

It would be inappropriate of me to go into the details of how it happened. Our stories overlap, but the story of her baby is not mine to tell. The thing to know about it is that (a) it didn't make me any more broody (I defy any woman to witness another woman's early pregnancy up close and think, hey, that looks fun! I should totally do that!) and (b) I wasn't bound by her decisions. In fact, in the event of trying for my own baby, an infantile strand of my personality deliberately wanted to make different ones, lest I be accused of copying. If we were going to do this thing separately and suffer the deprivations of single parenthood, we might as well realize all the advantages, too—in my case, starting from scratch and doing precisely what suited me and my notional baby.

ALL I HAD to do was figure out what that was. For example, would I use a friend as a sperm donor, or a stranger? If the former, who? If the latter, how would I go about making that choice? Would I move back to London to try to wangle free treatment on the NHS? (Which, to the horror of the right-wing press, now offers fertility services to single women and lesbians—or LESBIANS, as per tabloid house style.) Or would I stay in America and spend tens of thousands on something that might not even work? How much was I willing to sacrifice to pay for this? My London apartment? My 401(k)? My shirt?

There was one question that, depending on the answer, might render all other questions moot, and that was whether I could even conceive. I suspected not. In most areas of my life I didn't feel particularly female and it seemed to me unlikely I would be successful in this, its purest biological expression, without a struggle. This was, perhaps, a weird assumption on my part; the idea that unless certain proprieties of being female are observed—a hunger for marriage; a willingness to take more effort with one's appearance than I was willing to take; an engagement with the question of whether women can or should "have it all," etc.—the rewards would be withheld. I wasn't ashamed of the situation in which I found myself as my late thirties approached, but I was ashamed of that lack of shame, which felt to me like a failure of femininity. And I felt shame about feeling this, too.

The thing to do, I had heard, was to get one's eggs counted. If I had only a few left, I'd better knuckle down and start thinking—really thinking, not shove-it-off-to-one-side-again thinking—about whether I had the gumption to do this. If there were dozens and dozens, I could shilly-shally about for a bit longer. The day before my thirty-seventh birthday and feeling tremendously organized—look at me! Consulting with doctors as a precautionary measure! I had practically had the baby already—I went to see an ob-gyn.

In London, if you need a doctor, you shuffle along to a local GP allocated by zip code, who, if you have a serious problem, refers you to a specialist. In New York, you go online, decide what's wrong with you, consult *New York* magazine's annual best doctors in New York list, ask friends and relatives for recommendations and, after finding the most expensive doctor approved by your insurer, ring his or her secretary to wheedle an appointment.

And then, my god, you pay for it. It's a source of bafflement to some Americans that Brits in the UK don't visit the doctor more often. How is it, American friends ask me, that given our free health care, we aren't constantly getting our thyroids checked or popping in for blood tests? It would never in a million years occur to a British person to go to the doctor to ask for a "mole map," for example, the anti–skin cancer protocol that those in New York who can afford it demand of their dermatologists at the start of every summer. (No one in Britain who isn't actively shedding layers has a dedicated dermatologist.) This is not, as Americans sometimes suppose, because of hospital waiting times or the "grubby" facilities, but because of how we regard our relationship with the NHS: not as that of client to service provider but of beneficiary to birthright. One of the first and most unnerving things I learned when I came to America was how to collude with my primary care physician against my insurers, just to get my claims through.

The ob-gyn came recommended by a hypochondriac friend whose referrals I take seriously and was exclusive, with a clinic on Park Avenue that felt like a private members club—all thick carpet and dim lighting, with an oil painting of a horse on the wall. After a fifteen-minute wait, I was shown into the consulting room, and a moment later a woman in her fifties swept in and began conducting the examination. Timidly, I asked her about counting my eggs.

"That's not something we do," she said briskly and looked at me as if I'd asked her to put on her hat and read the television news.

"I'm thirty-seven tomorrow. Shouldn't I be panicking?" I felt ridiculous, like a made-up case study in a women's magazine article.

"Not at all." She paused. Then she asked me kindly about my work, my life and my plans for the future while I mumbled noncommittal responses.

"I don't think you have to start worrying about this issue for at least another year," she said and smiled in a way that struck me as reassuring at the time, but that I suspected I might look back upon with mixed feelings, like the record of the Red Cross during World War II.

"She's crazy," I said to friends afterward—everyone knows you have to hit the panic button at thirty-five—and then I found myself thinking, well, if a doctor says it's OK to wait, it must be true. (That's another thing about the British; we never seek second opinions. Our personalities aren't set up for it.) And I liked her for trying to counter the general hysteria around female fertility. I thought—I knew—she was probably wrong, but I appreciated her for trying.

At the desk on the way out, I handed over my credit card to pay the $380 bill.

"Can I give you chlamydia?" said the receptionist.

"Um. Can it not be an STD?"

"Fine. Yeast infection?"

"Perfect."

She filled in the code for my insurers, signed the form, stamped it and handed it back to me, smiling.

"See you in twelve months."

Over the next ten months, I did a lot of things. I handed in my book. I went on vacation with L to Puerto Rico. I doubled my output for my newspaper. One night, at a bar in Midtown, I jokily asked my friend Dan, "Hey, wanna be my baby-daddy?" ("Sure," said Dan, and the next day sent me a computer-generated image of a baby's face made up of our two faces, plus our friend Sarah's, plus Hitler's.) Apart from that, the most I could manage was to look through my fingers at a few sperm bank Web sites, then stare at the wall in despair. On good days, going ahead with the baby plan felt like a foregone conclusion. On other days, it struck me as an impossibility up there with climbing Everest or shouting out random words on the subway. Meanwhile, my thirty-eighth birthday loomed and panic rose around me like the skirts on a Hovercraft.

Toward the end of 2013, I went on a series of book tours, first to South Africa, then around the United States, finally winding up at the book festival in Edinburgh, where Rosemary and I order one last round from the waiter, whose contemptuous politeness suggests we are more drunk than we think. And it is now, a few hours before dawn, that we get to the heart of the matter. Rosemary is adopted and has a better understanding than most of the shallowness of the debate around nature versus nurture. Even so, in the dying embers of our evening together, she and I fixate on what everyone fixates on in the early days of considering having a child via some kind of donor: not what people will say or think; not even whether it will work; but what the kid will look or act like if it doesn't look or act like us. What happens if, thirty years down the line, a stranger's genes surface and I find I've produced someone I don't recognize from the way I have raised them?

"What's the nightmare?" says Rosemary.

"Merchant banker," I say. "You?"

There is a long, thoughtful pause. "Tory Christian," she says.

TWO

Origin
Story

MY MOTHER had me a month shy of her forty-third birthday, a jaunty move in 1975. She was in good nick—five foot nine, slender, could pass for ten years younger and did, until I found her passport one day when I was about ten years old. "I thought you'd figured that out long ago," she said breezily, as if I'd come tragically late to the party, but I know it bothered her. "Older mothers make very good mothers," she would later say, somewhat sadly and echoing what the obstetrician at the Hammersmith Hospital had told her. "They just sometimes run out of steam."

It was a source of sorrow to my mother that she didn't have more children, such a rare admission of regret on her part that to me, growing up, it put motherhood in a singular category: as one of the few things you couldn't get for yourself via hard work or enterprise. It also left me with the impression that I might have trouble conceiving. By the time I was in my twenties, it was clear to me, even without my mother's example, that the way women like me had kids was at forty-three after three rounds of IVF, two on the NHS, one in the private wing of UCH, before scaling down their jobs to three days a week and leaving the office at six p.m. on the dot, so that two thirds of the population around them—the men, the young people, the women without children—resented them for not doing their share. As a punishment, they were forced to talk about work/life balance for the next twenty years, a debate so boring one might forestall having children just to avoid it.

And of course that's if they could get pregnant at all. I remember an older woman in my office who'd had a child in her late thirties and been unable to have more going on an impassioned rant to me about how women my age had been sold a lie; how all those you-go-girl pieces in the magazines about women having kids in their forties downplayed the sheer size of their gamble. I thought she was mad. Having "only" one child sounded fine to me, but in any case, I could barely imagine being thirty, let alone forty. The only thing I couldn't work out was this: after the amazing two decades I was about to have working and traveling and writing books and learning about myself, what if I didn't "meet the right person"?

You might think that a story about the path to single motherhood would list all the exes I burned through, the ones who got away, whom I should've or could've had kids with but didn't. Instead, my emotional life in my twenties and early thirties was arranged almost entirely around my friends, with the mushroom cloud of my mother's death in the middle of it and interrupted by my move to America. For a long time, I couldn't even decide if I was primarily dating men or women. I spent a lot of demoralizing nights out trying to work out if he was boring me because he was boring or if he was boring me because he was male. (Looking back, it was often both.) "What did you like about him?" friends would say the morning after I'd been out on a date, and I would have to think hard. "I liked his gray cashmere sweater."

Eventually, after an unhappy period of kicking people out in the middle of the night and generally messing around every single man I went out with—apologies in particular to the visiting student from Cambridge, whom, after he'd traveled for three hours on a bus to have dinner with me, I ejected at two a.m. on the coldest night of the year because I couldn't bear to wake up with him—I came to a reckoning: that while I can find men attractive, and even date them for a while, I'm much better suited sexually and emotionally to relationships with women. (If this can be rationalized, which it probably can't, I think it's because women are less romantic and more pragmatic than men, although it amuses me to note that things I would find insufferable in a male date—gold Rolex, sports car, an obsession with SoulCycle—I will admire in a woman as the fruits of empowerment. It's possible my feminism has a way to go yet.)

The larger point is this: even though, by the late 1990s, the feminist pendulum had swung away from an emphasis on self-sufficiency and back toward the equality of choice—specifically, a woman's right to choose to stay home with her kids and not be judged wanting by her feminist peers—my female friends and I all knew that some choices were more equal than others. Sex, marriage, motherhood, all mattered; they just didn't matter until they mattered. In the meantime, I was like every other self-respecting twentysomething woman who'd read Cixous at college and secretly rooted for Sigourney Weaver's character in *Working Girl*. I got my kicks at work.

. . .

WHEN I GRADUATED from college in 1997, the only people I knew my age who were in a position to have children were old school friends who hadn't moved to London after university but had returned home, married to their college sweethearts, having missed the memo that our generation of women didn't have to do that anymore. We regarded them with scorn; those who can, do, we thought, those who can't, breed. Fifteen years later these people would have their revenge: those who can, breed, those who can't, are screwed. But it didn't feel like that yet. At twenty-two, it felt like this period would go on forever.

I had graduated wanting to write for a living and made a list with the *Guardian* at the top and two trade papers, *Cage and Aviary Birds* and *Metal Bulletin,* at the bottom. I still half wish I'd had the chance to write about metals or birds. (I had a fantasy about becoming the first breakout star of avian journalism, in which my stunning piece about parakeets caught the eye of a national newspaper editor and vaulted me to the big time.) Instead, I went to Edinburgh to take up a job at the *Scotsman,* the national newspaper of Scotland, run by English people whom the Scots on staff hated and housed in a scruffy building on North Bridge that is now a boutique hotel. I was the youngest on staff and also the worst dressed. Of the three pairs of trousers I owned, one of them was made of brown leather.

Years later, when I came to consider having a baby alone, one of the phrases that ran through my head was "The meaning of life is three phone calls away." It was something an executive from News International had told me during a careers day at college, and although she was being glib—a useful mind-set in the field, it transpired—it stayed with me because it turned out broadly to be true. Journalists may or may not be the smartest guys in the room. They may be able to write, or not, speak other languages or not. They rarely get rich unless they go into management or move sideways into TV and they are often disheveled and socially inept. What they do understand, perhaps better than anyone, is that there is no defense that can't be breached if you hammer it hard enough or find a sly enough angle of entry. It was one of my mother's longstanding convictions that she would lose me in a kidnapping, and I sometimes think my entire career has been an effort to put myself in a room full of people who, when the masked men finally come for me, will know which three phone calls to make to get me out again.

In those early days in Scotland, not only did I have no idea whom to call, I had no idea whom to call to find out whom to call. I didn't know what any of the government agencies were called or how to extract official comment from them. I didn't know the difference between the civil service and the civil list. I was forever being told to get in touch with a celebrity and had no idea how one went about doing it, and when I did finally did get hold of one, I had no idea how to bring up the matter of their cosmetic surgery/conviction for shoplifting/terrible new film without getting thrown out of the interview. On my third day in the job, I was put in a cab and told to doorstep the wife of a cabinet minister who'd left her for his secretary. ("Why don't you leave her alone?" said the cab driver when I gave him the address. "She's already had some dickhead from the *Sun* climbing up her drain pipe this morning." And he left me in a downpour, outside her house in a suburb of Edinburgh, trembling with fear and ignorance.) I think I'd have been happier if she'd slammed the door in my face. Instead, after I stammered out a question that managed to avoid the words "husband," "secretary" and "affair," she looked at me with a sort of withering compassion and shut the door slowly. My leather trousers took three days to dry out.

For the next two months, between the hours of ten a.m. and six p.m. daily, I ran around Scotland chasing the requisite two case studies per story of people who'd had threesomes; nightclub bouncers on drugs; people who didn't let their kids watch TV; anorexics; bulimics; alcoholics; amputees; victims of prison rape; ex-SAS men turned mercenaries; Americans living in Scotland who'd had bad dental work; "anyone from the Buccleuch family" (Scotland's biggest landowners); tax avoiders; Masons; celebrity chefs; expert witnesses who'd been discredited at trial; women addicted to tanning machines; Scotland's oldest mothers, Scotland's youngest mothers, Scotland's surrogate mothers, Scotland's lesbian mothers, mothers of triplets, women who'd had multiple miscarriages; adoptees reunited with their birth families for the first time who would let me sit in on the meeting; people who lived on boats, in tents, in council houses marked for demolition. In my desperation, I learned the value of calling people at random from the phone book or stopping them in the street—"Hi, sorry, I know this sounds really weird, but you don't happen to know someone who stepped on a land mine and survived, do you? I can't pay them but I can buy them a drink"—or going round the back of the office to the pub, one of those hard-core drinking dens where from twelve p.m. onward there was always someone drunk enough to spill the beans on himself or refer me to someone whose category of trauma matched the thing I was looking for.

I learned that if you look demoralized enough, people will take pity on you and help, and that being a woman assists with this, not because they think you are stupid, but because they think you are harmless. When, at the end of this period, I got a job at the *Guardian,* the terror of not knowing what I was doing had been replaced by the slightly less debilitating fear of simply doing it badly.

The *Guardian* was supposed to be a step up, about as far from the tabloid-management style of the *Scotsman* as you could get this side of the *Church Times*. It was the newspaper my parents had read until they switched to the *Independent* because, said my mother, there was something wrong with the *Guardian*'s printing presses and too much ink came off on her fingers. At the *Guardian,* no one came out of their office at six p.m. to shout and wave their arms around. No one ever threw a punch in the newsroom or called anyone else a cunt, at least not to their face. And although the lead times were short, they weren't *that* short. At college, I had done all my essays under self-imposed exam conditions, in three hours flat before my weekly tutorial, and I was starting to wonder if I might be one of those people who can function only under pain of a tight deadline.

The main thing about the *Guardian* in those days is that its outward appearance was as shambolic as its inner workings. Under every desk was a mountain of unwashed sports gear piled high on a bank of overloaded power outlets on top of which, inevitably, rested someone's rank sneaker. Decades' worth of cutting files and press releases towered on every surface until the inevitable landslide occurred. It was often speculated that a kind of slow-mo Pompeii was taking place so that one day years into the future, archaeologists would dig us all out from a bedrock of twenty-five-year-old book galleys and unused invitations to Internet 1.0 launch parties. After I moved to New York, I visited a friend at the *Wall Street Journal* and didn't recognize a newsroom in which someone wasn't doing magic tricks in the corner, or pretending to answer the phone as if it were the Communist daily—"Hello, *Morning Star?*"—or standing at his desk in his boxer shorts while changing for racquetball, or playing practical jokes that resulted in the evacuation of the entire building, all of which, in the world of American journalism, would trigger the swift and decisive involvement of HR.

Six weeks into my job, Ian, my editor, dumped a stack of papers on my desk. "Read these and pick a winner," he said. Most of the entrants for Student Journalist of the Year were long, terrible disquisitions about what the twenty-year-old in question thought should happen in the Middle East and which, at twenty-three, I personally found very juvenile. One stood out; a girl from Manchester University who'd written about schoolkids trying out for Manchester United. It was well researched, well written and well structured. "This one," I said. Merope was eighteen months my junior, and twenty years later, she still takes it half in good spirit and half in irritation when I remind her that she owes everything to me.

The years that followed can be visualized as a north London version of *The West Wing,* only with no budget for wardrobe and dialogue that revolved exclusively around where to have lunch. We arrived late and left late. We called one another on the way to the office, spent all day talking, had lunch together and talked all the way home. One day, a man with a large head took the seat opposite mine. Oliver was my age and had just graduated from Cambridge, and while he was neater than me and would push back the rising tide from my desk daily, in most other respects we aligned. On the wall above our desks, we affixed what were, we agreed, the two greatest tabloid headlines of all time—An Old Woman Beat Me for Being a Drunk When in Fact I Was Having a SEIZURE and A Careless Moment at a Garden Bonfire and Engelbert Humperdinck's Son Was Engulfed in Flames—and began a conversation that is still going strong.

Years later, a British friend who worked at a newspaper with a less cultlike nature and who got married at thirty and had kids like a normal person looked at me quizzically over drinks in New York. "What was wrong with you all?" she said. She didn't mean this unkindly and I didn't take it as such. I knew what she meant. She meant why were we all single for so many years? Throughout our twenties, when you're sup-posed to be out having the romantic time of your life, figuring out who you like and don't like, getting all the mistakes out of the way prior to settling down, we were at our desks until late or getting pissed at The Coach and Horses then calling one another on the way home to discuss where pigeons go at night, or what it's like to work at the top of a crane, or to get "closure" on something someone had said to us that day, or to ask, with complete sincerity, "Hey, did we ever talk about time travel?" or simply to state, on the basis that the more trivial the observation, the greater the testament to the friendship, "We had lunch."

Occasionally, someone had sex, but it was rarely a good experience. Merope had a thing with someone in her building to whom we all hi-lariously referred as her "sex-door neighbor." Oliver went on some dates with a woman we called, for reasons I forget, "the tea lady." I became briefly obsessed with a low-grade narcissist, who after a few weeks thankfully threw me over for another victim. Our friend Leila actually lived with someone for a few years, but it didn't work out, so she went back to seeing a guy she went to college with who'd come over on a Friday night and not leave her flat until Sunday. It was during this era that I got into a bad habit of treating dates like any other kind of un-promising material, so that when a man I'd been out with a few times told me about the death of his father, I dropped my head to one side and, to his apparent gratification and my enduring shame, said, "How did that change you?" I went on three dates with a nice but dull man in advertising, and when my colleagues found out they got his address from the electoral role and told me they'd sent him flowers on my be-half. (They hadn't.) Everything was grist, nothing was sacred. In this way our twenties played out.

Even when the sex-door neighbor was shelved and Merope got a se-rious boyfriend, nothing much changed. On her twenty-sixth birthday, it didn't occur to Oliver and me for a moment that it might be intrusive to turn up on her doorstep at eight a.m. with coffee and croissants. "HELLO!" we shouted, cramming our heads round the door, while from the stairs her boyfriend gave a wan smile and a wave as Merope barged past him to let us in. We were ambitious and loved our jobs, about which, like most journalists, we had an inflated sense of impor-tance, but looking back, the simple explanation for all this is that we loved one another. When we talked about the long-range future it was to joke that one day we'd all end up in the mythical Old People's Home for Journalists in Devon and wouldn't that be lovely. There were never any husbands or wives in these scenarios, although I think we all as-sumed that at some point we'd have to knuckle down and sort out our personal lives. In the meantime, the image we had in our heads was of us, our friends, our editors, all old together, doing exactly what we were doing then, but with shorter hours and longer deadlines.

And then something terrible happened, something truly catastrophic. Merope got pregnant. The marriage she, Oliver and I had been in for eight years, in which we referred to one another as our "outboard brain" and took it as read that if one said to another "Don't tell anyone else" it didn't apply to the absent third party, was blown apart. Her boyfriend drove her to my house for crisis talks and waited in the car beneath my living room window. Merope and I stood there, like something out of a 1960s kitchen sink drama, my laundry on a drying rack in the middle of the room, fridge empty save for a can of Coke and some mushrooms. Even as my heart broke, I felt very strongly what a good thing this would be for her. A baby! Of course she should have a baby. Come to think of it—and I hadn't thought about it much before then—everyone should have a baby. Shit, I should have a baby, not then, obviously, but at some point. A surge of panic shot through my system. How, I wondered, would I ever have a baby when I couldn't stand to see anyone for more than three dates and was tipping away from men toward women?

"I just thought I'd have you for longer," I said.

"Don't say that," said Merope. And we both wept.

This was, of course, a love scene but we weren't in love like that, although I know people occasionally wondered. And looking back, it is absurd to think that a twenty-nine-year-old woman having a baby with her boyfriend-soon-to-be-husband should have been received by our social group as so shocking. But women like us had our babies at forty, not twenty-nine, and she might have been a teen mother for the scandal it caused.

Overnight, Merope's pregnancy exposed the limitations of our lives, which seemed suddenly juvenile and small. I had always assumed that when it came to having babies, I'd make my three phone calls and figure it out, but faced with Merope's concrete example, that plan—or lack of a plan, as it now appeared—seemed unrealistic. And while, throughout my twenties, I had been confident there was no fate worse than being married with kids and moving to the suburbs, now a fresh nightmare floated to mind: that of being a single forty-year-old woman sitting in the same chair at the *Guardian* that I had occupied since the age of twenty-three. A person could grow old and bitter and unhappy if she put too much investment in her identity as it pertained to her news organization, not because it was "only" a job, but because, as Merope's defection made clear, it wasn't the only job. Not long after the announcement, she went on a Scandinavian cruise with her boyfriend and kept her phone off the entire time.

And so I did something rash, partly driven by my ambition to avoid sitting in the same chair for the next ten years, partly because, at the age of thirty, I thought if I didn't act immediately nothing interesting would ever happen to me again, and partly in a fit of petulant fury that my best friend had upped and got pregnant, with a man, of all things.

"Is it because I'm pregnant?" said Merope miserably when I told her I was resigning and moving to America. I replied with all the grace and temperance of someone unexpectedly confronted with an unpleasant truth about themselves: "That is fucking unbelievably insulting, it's not ABOUT you, how DARE you." And we both cried again.

It took a few weeks to get the juice up to act, and when I did, it was on the morning I'd had three fillings at the dentist and was as high as a kite on the drugs. Right, I thought, marching back up the Aldgate to the office. Let's do this thing. When I got in, I sent an e-mail to the editor's secretary asking for a meeting, and an hour later told him I was resigning my staff job to move to America. I had no plan, nowhere to live and a single friend in New York, but I had a four-year visa, and because I went there every five minutes for work, I figured it was just about doable.

Alan went through the formal motions of offering me incentives to stay. "Do you want to go to Iraq?" he said mildly, which might seem like an odd offer, but war reporting, the noble end of my profession, is something toward which we are all at some level assumed to aspire. "No, thanks," I said and sketched out an idea for him I had of freelance life that involved working for three weeks in New York, then going to sit on a beach in Mexico for two, and which, looking back, makes me wonder at the strength of the drugs I'd been given.

Alan said something generous then, that even as I shook at the thought that I was doing the wrong thing—that I was jacking in a job I would have killed for ten years earlier—made me feel I'd be all right and wouldn't die obscure, alone and broke, far from home. He said, "I envy you."

A few months later, I served my last day, and a week after that, Merope, Oliver and I went on a valedictory trip to Ireland, during which it rained the whole time and we bickered about one another's map-reading and driving skills. A few days later, the news editor, who had known us both for ten years, clicked her fingers at Merope and said teasingly, "Are you the one who's pregnant or the one who's going to America?" Merope related this to me on the phone a week later, by which time I was standing on the thirty-sixth floor of a Manhattan sky-scraper, looking out toward New Jersey and this terrible mistake I'd made, my new life.

I HAD GROWN UP with my mother's stories of how it was to emigrate from Johannesburg to London; the coldness of that first winter; the unremitting coldness of the English; the disappointments of reality when held up against a dream. None of this had seemed relevant when I moved to the United States. After all, our circumstances were completely different. She had arrived in England at the age of twenty-seven, unemployed with scant savings and with nowhere to live after her week in the hostel ran out. When I moved to New York at thirty-one, it was to a job and an apartment. (The gods of fertility are capricious, heaven knows, but they are nothing compared with the gods of New York real estate, and before moving I had been blessed with a bona fide miracle—a below-market one-bedroom on the Upper West Side.) South Africans in London were regarded as lowly colonials; Brits in New York clung to the last vestiges of a national superiority complex. And while it took my mother three weeks to get to England by ship and seven years to save up the money to go back, I arrived at JFK after the usual seven-hour flight and went home for my first visit a pathetic three weeks later.

And yet a few weeks in and in spite of all this, I was searingly, savagely lonely.

I could go into great detail about those early days, the experience of moving somewhere for broadly cinematic reasons and then having to deal with the reality. Suffice it to say that, just as my mother had discovered, in 1960, that living in London was not like a montage of scenes from *Waterloo Bridge, A Tale of Two Cities* and *A Nightingale Sang in Berkeley Square,* forty years later I learned that life in New York is a little flat without the Carly Simon soundtrack.

The answer, said my colleague Ed, a British immigrant of several years' standing, was to "say yes to everything," as a result of which I went to a lot of roof parties in Bushwick and club nights on the Lower East Side, including one called Ass Wednesday, at which a man in a leather thong shook his booty in my face while I tried to reach around him for bar snacks. I went to events at the British consulate and dark bars in which people read aloud from their unpublished novels. I even made a desultory effort to date in those first few months, trying to summon the same cavalier attitude I'd had in London and laugh it off when a man invited me to his loft, showed me his gun collection and a week later blanked me at a party at the *Paris Review.* Another, a banker friend of a friend, seemed to be laboring under the delusion that I'd won first prize in a competition to spend two hours auditioning for a part in his future. I went on lots of dates with passive-aggressive vegan women who did yoga and had strong views about bike lanes. But without my friends to discuss it with the following morning, these vignettes stopped being funny and started being depressing.

A few weeks after I arrived, Merope's baby was born.

"She's fucking cute," said Merope on the phone from London. She sounded fierce, almost angry, not a tone of voice I'd heard her use before.

"What was it like, seeing her for the first time?" I said meekly.

"It was like being punched in the face by love."

This sounds gilded, I know, but she really did say it. My heart sank. I thought of my recent slew of disastrous dates and consoled myself with the thought that I was only thirty-one and in America—America!—where it is practically unconstitutional not to get what you want. The fact is, I'd half been hoping Merope would say, nah, it's rubbish having a baby, you can strike it off your to-do list and get on with the rest of your life.

Two months after arriving, I moved out of the skyscraper to a regular apartment downtown. A few weeks after that, I went to a Sunday brunch organized by friends of my cousin and met Dan, an editor at an entertainment magazine, who I knew was on my wavelength when he referred to the Freedom Tower as the Infidel Trade Center and on the walk home stopped dead in the street to look up at a branch and observe, "Wow, I've never actually seen a pigeon pooping before." I met Sarah, a writer, at the birthday party of a mutual friend, and after introducing her to Dan, a new gang was born. A few weeks after that, Oliver moved to DC to cover the general election and by the following year was living in Brooklyn.

Meeting L wasn't a matter of thunderbolts. It was quieter than that, more surprising; the realization that love can be as simple as having someone see through you without running away. On the phone with her one night not long after we met, I started asking lots of intense questions about her childhood. About her family, and her childhood pet, and the time she got thrown out of French class for repeatedly saying *"oui-oui."*

"But were you just trying to be funny or were you trying to get thrown out?" I said, then asked four further follow-ups. On and on I went until eventually she burst out laughing. "Are you *interviewing* me?!" she said.

WRITERS BABY OTHER WRITERS; nonwriters don't, not because they don't care but because they don't understand how feeble we are in the face of even the mildest criticism. A year later, when I plucked up the courage to give L a draft of my book, she read it on the bed in her apartment on the Upper West Side, while I lay beside her curled up like a shrimp. "There," she said, pointing over her pregnant belly to a passage about my mother's late sister, a woman I had found extraordinarily difficult. "And there." L read the passage again and turned to look at me critically. "Why are you being so cheap with the reader? Why don't you say what you feel?" I felt like I was standing in the beam of a searchlight.

I had imagined that finishing the book might clarify things between us. Then I'd thought that L's pregnancy would surely change things one way or another. I had supported her efforts to get pregnant, but it had been hard and weird, and in the months after she conceived, I was sick with envy, not of the pregnancy itself—the three-year age gap between us had never felt more pronounced—but of the attention she received, and of the women with children whose advice she sought over mine. When the baby arrived, I was sure that *that* would finally throw some evolutionary switch and we would automatically know what to do. But that didn't happen, either. I carried on spending three nights a week and all weekend at L's apartment, and the rest of my time at home or traveling for work. It shamed me sometimes how relieved I felt to walk away from the stress and the crying and go home to my quiet apartment in Brooklyn.

A male friend once complained to me about feeling pushed out in the delivery room, setting the tone, he said bitterly, for the entire parenting enterprise. I had thought this pitiful at the time. That's rich, I thought. Typical man, doing less of the child care then complaining about feeling pushed out. But now I felt the same way. Worse, in fact, because I had no designated role. If I felt "pushed out," pushed out from what, exactly? And yet neither of us wanted to move closer in.

When the baby was six weeks old, my book launched in the United States. L persuaded a friend of hers to lend me her art gallery, found a supplier for the champagne, swelled the guest list by inviting her out-of-town cousins, and on the afternoon before the party, she stood in her kitchen with the baby strapped to her front and made cucumber sandwiches for seventy. At five a.m. the next morning, a car took me to the airport to fly to South Africa. For the next fortnight, I talked exclusively about my mother. I talked about how funny she was, how good, and kind, how impatient of weakness. I talked about how much she loved me. I told all the stories she had never told me herself: about how she had had her father, the child molester, arrested and brought to trial for abusing his children; about how the trial had collapsed and she'd left South Africa, almost never to return. Over and over I said these things, to South African women who looked and sounded like my mother, tough old boots who came up to me after events and said "That's my story, too" in a way that made me wonder where they had buried the bodies. My mother believed that the only guaranteed love in a life is for one's child, on whose account another adult might be loved, loathed or simply tolerated, but who would never come close to being loved the same way. I realized I believed in this the way I believe in sunlight and air.

When I got back from South Africa, I almost immediately went on another book tour in the United States. In a bookstore in Boston, a woman stood up and, covering her mouth with her hand, said shyly, "I don't usually wish ill on anyone, but I heard recently that my abuser died." She removed her hand to reveal a broad smile. "I was so happy." The entire room burst into applause.

There was one story I didn't tell on publicity tour. It was about a cousin of mine, a few years older than me, who ten years earlier had been on the brink of marrying a man she wasn't sure about. A few months before the wedding, she had come to stay at my parents' home in Buckinghamshire. It was the summer my mother was dying and I was living at home, periodically traveling up to London to show my face at work, then hurrying back on the train, sick with dread at what I might find.

My cousin's mother was long dead, and although she didn't know my own mother well, she asked her for advice about the wedding. My mother was woozy on drugs and secondary brain cancer by then but she suddenly became as sharp as a pin. "Do you want a child?" she said, leaning forward in her chair and fixing the younger woman with a ferocious look I knew well.

"Yes," said my cousin. "Very much so."

"Well, then," said my mother. "You must do whatever is necessary." And she sank, exhausted, back into her chair.

The absences from L and the baby were hard. I missed them, not with the acute longing with which I would one day miss my own children while traveling, but with a deep sense of connection I hadn't experienced before. I rang as often as I could, from hotels and airports, and was relieved at the end of the summer to fly to Edinburgh for the last event in my schedule. When I got to the hotel, I opened the suitcase to find that L had placed, without my knowledge, a tiny clean diaper on top of my clothes. I sat on the bed and burst into tears.

When I got back to Brooklyn, it was to a familiar feeling of relief that my travels were over and of not yet quite being home. I could never figure out what I was homesick for in these moments. Not for my flat in north London, nor for my dad's house in west London, where he had moved a few years after my mother's death. It wasn't for L and the baby, either. I had missed them enormously, but even the anticipation of seeing them the next day didn't altogether staunch my unease. Home is where the mum is, I thought stubbornly, a childish mantra that had run through my head ever since my own mother's death. As I stood in my living room in the late afternoon light, staring at my books and my furniture, at the painting done for me by friend Alexis that, although she swore this wasn't her intention, looked like an abstract of the Virgin Mary and child, this phrase drummed through my mind with new urgency. My eye fell on some cheap pink plastic shot glasses left out on the counter. Someone had given them to me for my thirtieth birthday and they had somehow made their way into one of the crates shipped from London. Home is where the mum is, home is where the mum is. Look at those, I thought vaguely; they would make good cups for a child having a tea party.

THREE

The Selfish Gene

CONCEIVING ALONE IS, by necessity, an inorganic process. There is no easing your way in by chucking out your contraception and six months later, if nothing has happened, sitting down with your partner and considering your options. Instead, one day you are going about your business as usual, the next you're crashing up against words like "treatment schedule," and "artificial insemination" and, most unhappily of all, "sperm donor," only to slam into retreat, like a boat trying to dock in bad weather. A million choices have to be made before you can get going and each choice feels as if it will result not only in a different person's being born but in an entirely different story of where that person has come from. I had thought the biggest barriers to having a baby alone would be physical and financial, but that fall, I encounter something that halts women in their tracks more surely in this situation than dwindling egg supplies or bad credit: a failure of imagination.

After the meeting with the ob-gyn on Park Avenue, I decided there was no point in getting my eggs counted until I knew what I was going to do with them, and so, one evening that fall, I head to an Italian restaurant in the Village to have dinner with friends, a no-nonsense couple who have managed to produce a startling three children from a combined parental age of around ninety. L doesn't come with me. In some ways, things are simpler between us than when she was trying to get pregnant; she already has her baby and is less inclined to feel threatened or excluded, as I did when the roles were reversed. But it's complicated, too. I don't know if I can get pregnant, and if I do get pregnant, I don't know if L and I can survive, and if we do survive, I don't know in what form that might take. But if, by some miracle, we ever do get to the point of—what even to call it? Parallel parenting? Proximal parenting? Parenting in each other's general direction?—the one thing that seems likely is that it will be harder for both of us if my decisions differ too wildly from hers.

"Hmph," she says, when I mention my friends.

"I'll let you know how it goes."

Like a lot of lesbian couples half a generation older than me, my friends conceived via what is mockingly referred to as the "turkey baster" method, an informal arrangement between parties at home, keeping costs down and, in countries with harsh fertility laws, allowing single women and lesbian couples to avoid the clinics and the interference of the state. Using a friend as a donor also offers the thinnest connective tissue to the conventional family. Everyone is better off in this scenario, it is said, because the child has an identifiable father and so "knows where it comes from."

At first, my friends go along with this. Yes, they say, it is reassuring to know who he is. No, of the two of them, the one who didn't give birth doesn't feel marginalized, although it took awhile for them to figure out the family dynamic. Yes, they tell me, the kids have contact with their father and derive something meaningful from that. The tone of the conversation becomes increasingly fraught and as more wine is brought out with the entrées, they crack.

"The truth is we hate him," says Rebecca.

"What?" I say.

"He's a fucking asshole," says Tanya. She says this with such vehemence the candle on the table flickers. It is, she says, tremendously difficult having a third wheel in the family, particularly one who, over the years, has asserted his connection to the children more and more aggressively. There are legal provisions in place to protect my friends' sovereignty as parents, but it is morally complicated, figuring out what access to give him and how much of his interference to tolerate.

"Shall we say it?" says Tanya, and looks at her wife.

"Go on, you say it," says Rebecca.

"OK," she says. There is a long pause. "We sometimes say that if it could be painless, and not hurt anyone, and if it wouldn't damage the kids, life would be better if he just . . . disappeared."

I know how this sounds. It's how a lot of women talk about their ex-husbands and is the source of much bitterness on the part of those men who feel their contributions to their children aren't adequately recognized. It also echoes something I am starting to hear from other people that fall; that increasingly in New York, ob-gyns are discouraging single women from conceiving with a friend in favor of using an anonymous donor. Emotionally, it's less complicated. You don't have to budget for a man setting eyes on the baby and reconsidering his resolution not to be involved. It can be easier for the mother, too; no matter how many times you tell yourself you are doing this alone, if there is an identifiable father, some lizard part of your brain will insist he should be helping. As for the argument that the child is better off knowing who the dad is, if he isn't available as a dad, it can potentially open the door to a lot of feelings of rejection.

All of this makes sense to me intellectually. But at dinner that night, I find myself thinking, well, my friends obviously chose badly. I wouldn't make the same mistake because my male friends aren't douche bags. A few months earlier, when I had asked Dan if he wanted to be my baby-daddy, I'd been more or less joking, but posing the question even flippantly felt like a form of due diligence. Didn't I owe my hypothetical child at least that, a stab at what, from the outside, looked like the more normal arrangement? Have a baby with someone you know and you might at a glance be divorced. You might simply have gotten drunk one night and hey presto. Or maybe you made one of those cute pacts between friends that form the basis of rom-coms, the ones in which college buddies determine that if they're both single and childless at thirty-eight, they'll go ahead and have a baby together. This is, obviously, very bad reasoning from the point of view of what psychologists would call owning your situation. But in spite of that fact, and in spite of knowing all the downsides—the possible unfairness to the friend, the logistical headache, the sense of ickiness that comes, one imagines, from two millennia of evolution bearing down on me for even thinking of having a baby with someone I'm not sexually attracted to—it still seems a lot less frightening than having a baby with a blank space.

There's an interview I keep thinking about that I did for my newspaper ten years ago. It was with a woman called Diane Blood, who had lobbied all the way to the House of Lords for the right to conceive using her dead husband's sperm. Stephen Blood had died of meningitis at the age of thirty, and while he was lying in a coma, his wife, Diane, had asked doctors if they could extract his sperm, so she could have his baby at some point down the line. They duly extracted the sperm and litigation began.

It was a complicated, unusual case that set a precedent unlikely to be much called upon, hinging as it did on the right of a surviving spouse to conceive using her dead partner's sperm, and to have the deceased's name put on the birth certificate. Blood was a ferocious campaigner, who, after a lengthy battle with the Human Fertilisation and Embryology Authority, finally won the right to take the sperm abroad for fertility treatment. She had two children by her late husband in this manner and succeeded in getting the law changed so that he was officially recognized as the father.

What still amazes me about this case is the level of vitriol directed at her. She was ridiculed in public. Religious people compared her baby with Dolly the sheep and accused her of assaulting her husband while he lay in a coma. The HFEA, in a moment of almost comical philosophical overreach, asked Blood *what her dead husband would have wanted,* the rights of a dead man apparently superseding those of his still-living wife. (Oddly, this was a question Blood was able to answer. By coincidence, she said, not long before her husband's death, they had come upon a magazine article about another woman wanting to have a child with her dead spouse and Stephen had said that in the event of his own death, she should go for it.) None of this satisfied the critics. The fact is, said a politician blithely on the radio one day, Blood's son "should never have been born," a remark she overheard while in the Neonatal Intensive Care Unit, where her premature baby lay fighting for his life. Ten years later, recounting the memory to me, she was still raw with the shock of that moment. "We are real people with real feelings," she said.

I was twenty-seven at the time of the interview and Blood was the age I was in the fall of 2013—thirty-seven—and although I was sympathetic to her in print, privately I remember thinking what a lot of people thought at the time: "ew." It was creepy. Why saddle your kids with that kind of legacy? She didn't deserve the abuse, of course—nobody did. But there was something mad about the enterprise, something fanatical. For god's sake, I thought; just how badly did this woman need children?

THE WORLD HAS MOVED ON since then and my circumstances are completely different from Blood's. At least—and there is always an "at least" in these scenarios—I'm not trying to have a child with a dead man. But as I try to move forward with my decision making that autumn, there it is, standing like a brick wall between me and the future: Ew. Gross. Ew. There are days when I feel shame in so many directions at once, I don't know what to avert my eyes from first. It is shameful to visit an absent parent on a child. It is shameful to look ahead at a childless future and be horrified. It is shameful to have the sneaking suspicion that in spite of the terribly hard things going it alone might entail, it will be easier than doing it with L. The very fact that I am considering going to these lengths in order to get pregnant must mean I want a baby to a much greater degree than I care to admit, and therefore that it might be a hard thing to unwant. And this is shameful, too.

Even my consolations are shameful. With any luck, I think, I'll squeak in with a baby just under forty (good!). But I am a single woman (bad!). I am in a relationship (good!). But we aren't doing this together (weird). Also, it is same sex (bad). On the other hand, a sperm donor is more "natural" than an egg donor, which is more "natural" than adoption, which is more "natural" than surrogacy, which is more "natural" than no children at all, a domino run that ends at the foot of the towering black tombstone marked "childless spinster." When a friend tells me about a woman she knows who used a service in which the sperm donor came round to her house and actually had sex with her, in a burlesque version of a "normal" relationship, I am over the moon. People might think what I'm doing is odd but that—*that*—is genuinely crazy.

I know these comparisons are spiteful. I also know that by focusing on them, I'm appealing for relief to the very thing that is causing me harm. Still I keep doing it. Moral superiority is quick and easy and it's kind of fun, too. Haven't we all, in low moments, reached for the comfort of despising other people and bolstered that need with stuff from the newspapers? Looking for something to be furious about? Not tempted by immigration, welfare queens, executive pay or the Middle East? Then how about an issue with bilateral appeal that has been reliably causing outrage for two thousand years—what women are doing with their bodies and how YOU can get involved!

Some easy points of entry:

Women who have only one child are selfish.

Women who have a child alone are selfish.

Women who don't have children: SELFISH, because—wait, how can not having children be selfish? Oh, right, because they have more time to lavish on themselves, flopping about on the sofa all day eating bonbons and never truly learning the meaning of self-sacrifice.

Women having children and then working full time: selfish.

Women having children, not working and expecting the taxpayer to foot the bill: selfish.

Women having children, not working and complaining that child care is so prohibitively expensive that it makes no sense for them to go back to work, even though they want to: selfish.

Women waiting until they are forty to have a child: selfish.

Women having a child at seventeen: selfish.

Women having an abortion: selfish.

Women having a child in the context of a same-sex relationship: self-ish. Also, gross. Come on. That's not what god intended. It's unnatural. (A couple of things on that point. Chemotherapy is unnatural. So is electricity, shampoo, air travel and five-a-side football. The hairpiece worn by the pastor is unnatural, as is the imitation-wood pulpit he clings to.)

And the mother of all selfish endeavors, the creation of a child using biotechnology. In the last thirty years, as IVF has become common-place, so the term "test-tube babies" has died out, to be replaced by the new pejorative, "designer babies," implying wanton use of fertility treat-ment and the choosing of things better left to chance or god's grace: hair and eye color, IQ, and the sex of your baby. Never mind that the majority of these things are neither legal nor in some cases possible, nor that, at most clinics in the West, you can't choose any of your baby's characteristics beyond the broad stroke of selecting an egg or a sperm donor, a choice as calculating as choosing a man with a Ph.D. from a dating Web site, or hitting on a guy with blond hair in a bar.

I have read references in the press to gay men having babies via sur-rogates as "consumer choice," as if their urge to reproduce isn't driven by the same primal impulse that strikes everyone who wants kids, but is instead an extension of the desire for accessories. That's what gay men do, right? For them, babies are just a higher-maintenance version of the Philippe Starck juicer.

Yes, says the Greek chorus, but what about love?

Shortly followed by: why don't you just adopt? (Or get a dog.)

And finally: say what you like, it still isn't normal.

It doesn't matter that my entire social circle is liberal. As anyone over the age of thirty who has ever been to a dinner party knows, parenting flushes out weird pockets of fanaticism in otherwise reasonable people. In Britain, something as simple as whether you choose to send your child to public or private school can make half your social group hate you, so that having a baby alone, or in the context of a same-sex relationship of indeterminate status, is likely to tip at least some of my peers over the edge.

I feel the first intimation of disapproval at dinner that night, when after asking me lots of questions about L—what we are doing, how we are doing it, why we aren't doing it differently, none of which I am able adequately to answer—I see my lesbian friends exchange glances. I know what they think. They think we are resisting merging households and becoming a nuclear family because of some internalized resistance to being "gay parents." Better to present as two single women helping each other out than as something from the pages of *My Two Mommies*. I give this some thought afterward—not much, but some—and wonder if L and I are not, as we believe, motivated by pragmatism and superior self-knowledge, but by some deep, homophobic self-loathing. Perhaps what we're doing isn't daringly modern, but actually depressingly retrograde. Then I think about the time we tried to put a bed from West Elm together and didn't speak for a week. I think about how unsuited we are to reaching mutual decisions. When the stakes are low—Indian or Chinese? Bridge or tunnel?—we can just about manage it, but it is hard to imagine either of us ceding to the other on the issue of what's best for a child. You can argue about the unfairness of this until the cows come home, but the fact remains: if, in most conventional families and even in progressive ones, there is typically a lead parent, the mother, and a deputy parent, the father, then two alpha mothers under one roof don't go.

·   ·   ·

OVER THE SUMMER, I had let my timetable slacken as I flew around promoting my book. Now, with the resolve that fall brings and the cost of fertility treatment potentially on the horizon, I say yes to every job that comes in. I interview people I've interviewed before. I interview people I know personally and shouldn't be interviewing. I interview supermodels and actors who have been repeating themselves for decades, jobs that would ordinarily depress me, but that now fill me with a martyrish purpose. Here I am, asking a movie star what attracted him to his role in *Speed Demon IV,* as a piece of bona fide self-sacrifice for my future child's diaper fund.

One of the jobs I say yes to involves a trip back to London to interview a British actor who is very au courant that season. We sit in a hot restaurant in Piccadilly, trying to ignore the stares of the other patrons while talking about his TV show. I ask him about his childhood and his acting training and his wife and family and then, to run down the clock and because it is the polite thing to do, he asks whether I have children. There is a school of thought—the right one—that in these circumstances the journalist should divulge nothing of herself and steer the conversation swiftly back to the interviewee. But it's a funny thing about famous people; I can say anything I like and, because journalists are to celebrities what PRs are to journalists—interchangeable units belonging to the world's most irritating subgroup of humanity—it will never, ever come back to haunt me, for the simple reason that five minutes after we part, he will have no idea who I am.

"My partner just had a baby but we're not doing it together," I blurt. He looks taken aback, briefly jolted out of his publicity setting. "Gosh," he says. "How does that work?" And so I tell him: about the dynamics of spending large amounts of time with someone who has a baby when I don't; about what it might mean if I have a baby of my own; about how I'm trying to decide how to do that. I say all this in a spritely tone quite at odds with the way I actually feel and that, even as I do it, I understand to be flirtatious in a way that is demeaning to both of us. From the outset, I believe it's important to be able to talk about all this, but this is not the same thing as knowing how to talk about it. "I don't know why you're interviewing me," says the actor when we part, "your own life sounds much more interesting!" not a line he believes and neither do I. Nobody wants an interesting personal life. Interesting is what you call it when you can't call it what you want to, which is messed up.

Something happens when I fly back to England from America: for the first few days, I continue to operate under the guise of my expat persona. I'm more impatient in line than a regular English person, more strident in the face of bad service. I don't send food back in restaurants, but I torment bus drivers by inviting them to have a nice day and generally present myself as someone aflame with efficiency, who has moved on from the sluggish ways of the old country. So it is that, after returning to my dad's house in west London after the interview, I pick up the phone to call Tessa. If anyone knows how to get me moving on this, Tessa will.

"Oh, darling, how fabulous of you!" she says, when I tell her I'm gearing up to follow in her footsteps. I'm sitting on my dad's bedroom floor with my back to the dresser and the landline—I only ever use a landline when I'm at my dad's—pressed to my ear while looking up at the room's assortment of furniture. My dad got rid of an awful lot when he downsized after my mother's death, but every room still contains at least one outsize piece—in this case a standing mirror in heavy dark wood—that if it fell on you would kill you. "Have you got a pen?" says

Tessa and gives me the number of a woman she says I should go to be-fore I do anything else.

"Will she count my eggs?" I say.

"What?"

"Nothing."

"She'll give you a blood test and a lot of advice. She's sort of a guru. She got me through my second pregnancy. And tell her you're a journal-ist; she might have media rates!"

Even though Tessa is the only person I know with older children conceived by anonymous donor, I don't ask her how things have turned out. I don't need reality right now, I need hope. I need cheerleading. I need someone to tell me, without judgment or caveat, that I can do this thing and it will all turn out OK.

OH, AND SPERM. I need sperm.

One of the things I'm discovering about making these decisions is that it is incredibly hard to be rational. I live in New York, but my emo-tional center of gravity still tilts toward home, and so, although it would be madness to choose a London-based donor, I reach for familiarity over practicality and, high on the spirit of Getting Things Done, after hang-ing up on Tessa call William.

I've been friends with William for fifteen-odd years and he's among the cleverest people I know, a former boy maths champion who is in the final year of a fast-track medical degree. He speaks passable Russian. He paraglides off cliffs. He has beautiful hands and wrists and a noble aquiline nose and green eyes and a sense of humor. Unlike almost every other man I know, he can distinguish one end of a wrench from the other.

I mention all this because, although we have never dated, in the days leading up to our dinner I find myself tailoring vignettes from our friendship into what can be described only as a romantic montage. A decade earlier, we had run up a huge tab at a horrible bar on Old Compton Street and tried to skip the bill, falling out of the door and running up the street doubled over with laughter. When I first moved to New York, William came to see me, went out drinking on his own and got in at three a.m. still wearing his suit, tie loosened and askew like a young Frank Sinatra. A year later, he diverted from a business trip to see me out in the Hamptons, swaggered across the deck like the hero in a bad Richard Gere film and threw himself into the lake, sending up a huge and not altogether flattering tidal wave. We have done a lot of boring, ordinary hanging out, too, but by the time I have finished editing these scenes, our friendship looks like something from *Breakfast at Tiffany's*— or rather from the movie *Green Card,* only the person I am trying to convince of our relationship isn't an immigration officer but myself.

What is this? I haven't, ten years into our friendship, suddenly contrived a deep-seated passion for William. Nor am I trying to talk myself into one. Instead, what I seem to be doing is shaping my memories to fit the backstory required of two people having a baby. I haven't even asked him yet and already, and without fully realizing it, I have gone from thinking of William as my cherished old friend to kitting him out as my charming ex-husband.

And haven't I done well! A soon-to-be doctor, brainy but strong, sensitive but practical, beautiful but brawny. This whole donor business flushes out some extraordinarily reactionary biases in me. Not only does William conform to 1950s standards of masculinity but—and this is the really insidious calculation—he is a good man, who if something were to go badly wrong with the baby would surely ignore everything I'd said about doing it alone and spontaneously leap to my rescue. This is why conceiving with friends can be such a bad idea: it opens the door to a lot of shoddy and treacherous thinking.

We meet in south London, at a basement Thai restaurant where most of the other diners are students, their bikes parked three deep at the railings outside, and where the paper tablecloths are spotted with wax from the tea lights. For the first hour, we catch up over spring rolls and noodles. William tells me about his recent breakup, the hell of being a student again and having no money, and how medical people are the pits with no social skills. I tell him about the publication of my book and my trip to South Africa, and about the joys and difficulties of being with L and the baby.

Toward the end of dinner, I say to William, "I have something to ask you."

"Oh, yes?"

I ask him.

"What do you think?" I say.

"I don't know. I did wonder if that's what this was about." He gives me a soppy look and takes my hand across the table, which I consider wonderful at the time but that looking back screams to me, BOUND-ARIES! "I'll have to think about it," he says. "But I'm pleased that you asked."

I don't tell anyone about my conversation with William. It feels too bizarre, too potentially shaming. These are early days, but I am discovering one of the unhappy truisms of the fertility world: that unless it's to a therapist (or a celebrity) people don't talk about it much, even if they're the kind of people who talk about everything. On any given day, I can open a newspaper and find someone I know writing about their depression, their waistline, their marathon training, their grief. When my mother died, I wrote a book about it. When my friend Alex moved from Britain to southern Italy, she wrote a book about it. When I return to New York from London, L asks how my friend Jake is after the death of his dad. "OK," I say. "He's thinking of writing a book about him."

"You people are gross," she says.

Actually, Jake is one of the few people whom I do talk to about it. He and his girlfriend have two kids, the first of whom took awhile to come along, so he has some experience of the world I am entering. A few days after my dinner with William I meet Jake at the South Bank, where we sit on benches outside the National Film Theatre, eating up-market kebabs from the van.

"It all sounds like a nightmare, I'm glad I'm not you," says Jake.

"Thanks."

"Why don't you and L just move in together and have a gaybie? Why are you being so selfish and weird?"

"We don't want to live together."

"Nobody wants to live together. You just have to do it."

"We don't. My baby doesn't have to be related to anyone I don't want it to be."

"What about"—Jake pauses to replenish the hot sauce on his sandwich—"the *dad*."

"It's not a dad, it's a donor."

"You could just clone yourself," he says. "Isn't that what you want anyway? Or have a baby with Oliver. Go on. It'd be hilarious. It'd come out of the womb arguing *with itself*. Hey, do you want my sperm? Actually, you can't have it. Emily wouldn't like it."

"You're too old. I don't want your old sperm."

"Yeah but"—Jake raises his eyebrows a couple of times, Groucho Marx style—"top-quality stuff."

"I'm sorry to have to tell you this, but I wouldn't touch your sperm with a ten-foot barge pole."

Look at me, I think later. Being all jaunty, avoiding the commonplace difficulties of marriage and children for something so much bigger and potentially more ruinous. Being with Jake lightens my mood and I feel suddenly quite giddy. I don't want to be "interesting" in the context of gossipy small talk, but there is a self-importance that comes with acting outside of the mainstream that after lunch with my friend, makes me preen and find myself almost unbearably fascinating. A few days later, when I turn up at the clinic of Tessa's guru in west London, I am still in high spirits.

They sink almost immediately. Seeking private health care in Britain feels illicit no matter the cause, as if one were cheating on the NHS, and the clinic, which is in a converted house that looks less like a doctor's office than one of the shabbier foreign embassies, makes me feel instantly shifty. The reception area is full of products stamped with the guru's photo, and when I pick up a leaflet I see that while it is advertised as an IVF clinic, a large number of the services have to do with counseling and nutrition.

One thing I have to be mindful of here is that what works for some people doesn't work for others and this woman's counsel obviously works for some people. Over the course of an hour's consultation, she says lots of sensible things about the stresses of trying to get pregnant. She asks about my moods and my objectives and my expectations of motherhood. When I try to explain to her that L and I aren't doing this together— that to us, stability and continuity mean loving each other, helping each other, maybe even raising our families alongside each other, while retaining the right to make independent decisions—she brushes it swiftly aside. No, no, no, she says. Before I choose a donor, or find a doctor, or do any of the things at the top of my to-do list, I have to Work On My Relationship. Conventional coupledom must be my ultimate goal. It'll be better for me, she says, and better for the baby. She is very firm about this. Single motherhood is hard enough, but not-quite-single-motherhood-we-don't-know-what-we're-doing is practically criminal.

I nod and agree. Through long professional habit, I have a very good poker face. I'm also highly suggestible. In the heat of the moment, there is almost nothing I won't agree to just to keep the person talking, and while the guru has the entire weight of Western thought about relationships behind her, all I have is my ambivalence and shame. Yes, of course. Conventional coupledom. That must be my goal. I must stop messing about and commit.

I had been thinking along these lines ever since my dinner with William, which I'd gone into leaning toward the view that a known donor is better than an anonymous one, and come out of less sure. William hadn't come back to me with an answer yet, but the encounter had left me uncomfortable. Something about it didn't feel right and now, as the guru lectures me, I think of our tender exchange at the candlelit dinner and feel queasy with guilt. What on earth am I doing, canoodling with William when I should be going all out to move closer to L?

"Relationships take work," says the guru and for a second our connection wavers. I've never been a fan of this axiom, which it seems to me is only ever directed at women as a reminder that large areas of their lives are going to suck and they needn't say they weren't warned. She looks at me expectantly.

"Right," I say. "No, you're absolutely right. We just need to work harder to figure it out."

. . .

I DON'T REMEMBER anything medical about my conversation with the guru. And while her tone is never less than sympathetic, afterward I see it as a throat-clearing exercise resting on vague assumptions of emotional disorder. The message seems clear; I am being at best perverse, at worst reckless. I had expected a clinical meeting about how to conceive. Instead, the whole thing felt like the prelude to a high-end backstreet abortion.

It was depressing for other reasons, too. I got a whiff of lifestyle evangelism from her, a sense that a large part of my success in getting pregnant would come down to a positive attitude and willingness to eat broccoli. I'm not against alternative treatments. During my mother's chemotherapy, Stoke Mandeville Hospital gave her free aromatherapy and reflexology and it was a lovely thing, a luxury and a break from the chemicals being pumped through her veins. But we were under no illusion that it did anything to alleviate the illness. We never got sucked into buying a juicer and trying to save her with pulverized cabbages, and the suggestion that these things work, for fertility as for cancer, makes me furious.

After the consultation, I hand over my credit card at reception, pay the £150 fee and walk down the street to the clinic's partner GP service, a private practice that feels even sadder and dodgier than the clinic itself and where, for another £150, a doctor gives me a blood test. A few days later, the results come back indicating that my hormone levels are on the low end of average for a woman my age, a finding that, without a treatment protocol in place, even I understand to be meaningless.

And that's it. Just like that I'm over the hump. All of this—my excruciating conversation with the actor, my dinner with William, the guru's advice, the nonsensical blood test—unite to trigger my Oh, For Goodness Sake reflex. I may not know what I want yet, but I know what I don't want. I don't want counseling and I don't want kale. I don't want another six months of hand wringing and I don't want whatever the guru is selling. What I want is to go back to America, a place that may not, ultimately, be the place I think of as home, but where the medical establishment is at least on my side. In Britain, as a single woman seeking a child, I am the subject of concerned official guideline and head-shaking dismay. In the United States, I am simply a consumer in a marketplace, not because I want a designer baby, but because that is how health care works, period, and for a short spell—a very short spell—this strikes me as the most wonderful thing in the world. In America, it's not for them to ask me questions, it's the other way round.

So, out I go and audition some doctors.

FOUR

Tubes

MY DAD IS NOT GIVEN to excessive displays of emotion. He is calm, reassuring, extremely measured about all things. Before he retired, he worked for forty years as a solicitor specializing in conveyancing, the least theatrical corner of the legal profession. The only subjects on which I have ever heard him voice an intemperate opinion are the filthy hot dog vans in central London, which he would like to firebomb, and Boris Johnson ("a toe rag"). Before leaving London, I do the one thing guaranteed to make my plan real; I mention it to him. Once you involve a parent, you open up a channel of concern and inquiry, a *drip drip drip* that it will be almost impossible to divert or fob off. It's like promising a toddler a treat; change your mind and you'd better have your story straight.

"So the plan is," I say, "that next year, or something like that, I'll do what L has done and try to get pregnant, because I'll be turning thirty-nine, time to crack on, makes sense if I want to have children, which I do, always have in fact, actually. Yup. So. That's."

We are on the road to Heathrow, driving around the southwest corner of Turnham Green just before Chiswick Town Hall. "Hmmm," says my dad, looking straight ahead.

I glance at him sideways. My dad is in favor of L because I am in favor of L, and also because he likes her. Along with Marion, my dad's partner, he has been enthusiastic about her baby. On the other hand, throwing a second baby into the mix without putting the relationship on a more formal footing is a challenging bit of news to absorb. My dad is liberal, but he is also a sixty-nine-year-old man who was married to my mum for thirty years. I wonder if even for him this mightn't be a step too far.

Nothing more is said about the baby that day, something that might worry me if I didn't know him so well. My dad has a habit of going quiet at the time of a major revelation, then chiming in later when he has had time to think. I know he'll be concerned about the logistics, not only of how I might cope alone with a baby, but of how I might cope alone with a baby so far from home. He'll wonder what my mother would have said and how she would have wanted him to respond. I smile as I consider this. The big gap in my mother's liberalism was around the raising of children; she was against people having kids outside of marriage. She thought pedophiles should be put to death or castrated. I don't recall us ever talking about gays having children—it wasn't around much as an issue in 1980s Buckinghamshire—but in spite of the fact that most of her best friends were gay men, my sense is she would have been disapproving. (In this she would, I think, have made a distinction between the suitability as parents of two men and two women.) For all her eccentricities, my mother idealized or even fetishized the traditional nuclear family, which she saw as a safeguard against the kind of childhood she suffered. On the other hand, she also saw it as her greatest achievement that I was free from that baggage and I have a feeling that, if I'd come to her with my plans that fall, she would have decided there and then that having a child alone, or in the context of an unconventional relationship, was the most brilliant thing any woman had done in world history. A few days after I get back to New York, my dad calls me at my desk in Brooklyn. "I've discussed it with Marion and we'll support you in whatever you do," he says.

CHOOSING A FERTILITY doctor is not like choosing a knee surgeon. If it was, you might simply browse a dozen clinic Web sites and pick the one with the highest success rate. Instead, when you meet a fertility doctor for the first time, you find yourself making all sorts of unscientific judgments. Do I like you? Do I approve of you? Do I want you to play a role in the story I tell about my kid's creation? Are we on the same wavelength so that my body doesn't go into spasms of dislike whenever it sees you and resists the tasks it is being asked to perform? All nonsense of course, otherwise no children would be conceived in bad relationships, but there you are. The dreadful woo-woo bullshit around fertility begins here.

"So how can I help you?" says the doctor. She is the first on my list, an ob-gyn with an office in Midtown who has come to me recommended by friends. I sit before her, legs crossed at the ankle, feeling like I'm on a first date and trying to revive my spirits after the experience of the waiting room, a tiny windowless space with an ornamental fountain that tinkled away like something designed to soothe the unnerved. The only other woman present was in an iron-gray suit and had very tightly curled hair. It described the atmosphere perfectly.

The doctor is in her late thirties, with big, sad eyes and an air of almost lascivious sympathy. Not my kind of doctor at all. In New York, my favorite doctor is Dr. Dolphin, my eye guy, who, sliding a needle into my lower lid one time, said, "Who's having more fun than you right now?! OK, heel to the steel!" (In the UK, my favorite doctor is the bluff, middle-aged woman GP who told me I did not, in fact, have stomach cancer, but had for years been wearing my jeans too tight.) This woman looks as if she were about to cry, and to overcome her piety, I crank my jocularity so high I sound like a seventies game show host. "Want to have a baby! . . . About to turn thirty-eight! . . . In a relationship but taking full moral and financial responsibility!"

She nods, unfazed by any of this, and after asking me a few general questions suggests we adjourn to the treatment room next door for the ultrasound. "Out of interest," I ask, gathering my things, "how old is the oldest client on your books?"

"Forty-seven," she says and adds quietly, "It's too old." I am so surprised by this candor that I feel myself warm to her, before realizing what I'm actually experiencing is a mean-spirited high from not being considered the worst-case scenario.

No one has ever looked at my ovaries before. No one has ever looked at my kidneys before, either, but kidneys are different, and as I climb onto the gurney, I find myself worrying about them on the basis that women worry about every other part of their anatomies: not that the doctor will discover something medically amiss, but that she'll hit upon some hitherto unrevealed ugliness. They could be misshapen, or asymmetrical or in the wrong place. They could be completely vacant, like one of those trick gift boxes that are empty save for a Christmas cracker–style joke. Perhaps all these years I've been sailing along thinking myself anatomically normal when, all the time, some twisted anomaly has been lurking within.

"Here," she says neutrally, and points to several dark patches. "Fibroids."

"OK."

She skims around a bit more, seeing things I can't see, then abruptly switches off the machine. "Very common, nothing to worry about, although we would keep an eye on them for growth."

This is the first and most superficial of a battery of tests that need to be done before treatment can start. My ovaries may look OK on the screen, but it remains to be seen if they're actually working, and to move on, says the doctor, there are more preliminaries—not, as in England, discussions about my emotions or lifestyle, but concerning something much more important: money. That is the real precursor to receiving medical treatment in the United States, and after the ultrasound, she ushers me through the waiting room into the office, for a meeting with someone far more significant than she is—the clinic manager—to talk about fee structure and financing.

Insurance anxiety is such a big part of this story it is worth pausing here to describe the lay of the land. My policy, which is administered in England and is available only to British nationals living abroad, is, with one very large caveat, absurdly generous by American standards. For the same price as the most punitive and exemption-ridden American policy, I have no deductibles, a co-pay of forty dollars per visit and, as far as I can tell from glancing at the small print, more or less limitless disbursements, so that in the years since moving to the United States, I have hammered it so mercilessly—endless checkups (it doesn't cover checkups, but every doctor I've been to has supplied the fake codes); multiple trips to Dr. Dolphin for recurring blocked tear ducts; an expensive biopsy on a lump of gristle in my right breast that a British doctor had deemed, on the basis of a manual exam, entirely harmless and that of course after thousands of dollars' worth of exploratory tests in New York, turned out to be so—that my dad jokes about selling his shares before I bankrupt the company.

A few days before my trip to the doctor, I had called my insurer's hotline in England, to see if they would cover my treatment.

"So, your husband—" said the operator. There was a pause, during which I could hear her belatedly engaging with the requirements of EU discrimination law. "In order to qualify for fertility treatment, your *partner* must also be a policy holder of at least two years' standing." Damn. Gender-neutral language. I had been all ready to bring up L and frighten them into approving me.

"What if there isn't one?" I said.

"I'm sorry?"

"What if I'm having a baby alone?"

"I . . ."

Static over the Atlantic. I felt sorry for her then; she was probably twenty-four years old and sitting in a cubicle in a business park in Slough.

"That wouldn't be covered by the terms of your policy," she said eventually.

"Can I ask why not?"

"I . . . it . . . I would have to . . ."

I could fight this. But the truth is, I don't really see why my insurers should pay for it. I understand that if the policy covers one type of person for treatment but not another, judgments are being made about who is deserving. And if they were denying me coverage on the basis of my sexuality, I would make all the necessary complaints. But either through moral cowardice or preemptive exhaustion at the thought of waging a futile battle, I have a tough time seeing "single woman" as a category that, in this instance, deserves equal protection under law. After all— and I have never articulated this to myself quite as clearly as I do in that moment—it isn't very respectable. It's selfish. I'm selfish. No more self-ish than anyone else wanting a baby, but to make a lifestyle choice that deviates so spectacularly from the norm and then expect other people to pay for it seems to me to be a bit bloody much. I get off the phone with a breezy "no problem," as if my inquiry had been entirely hypothetical, and think, maybe it's better this way. If it is going to be hard, let it be hard from the outset so I have time to muscle up and adjust. Insurance be damned, I'll pay for it myself.

The truth is I'm not yet worried about the cost of all this. I'm almost forty. I have a lot of savings. I've never spent more than I earn. I own property in one of the most valuable markets in the world. I think of all this, rather vainly, as being "sensible about money," although it has more to do with having (in English terms) a middle-class background, with all the safety nets and security that brings. A lot of outlandish things would have to happen—having more than one baby, say, or the economics of the entire news media falling into a hole or Britain's deciding to leave the EU, wiping a third of the value off sterling, none of which, obviously, is going to happen—before my assets start to dwindle. Looking ahead, I even relish the prospect of a little financial pain; it will reboot my ambition, I think, make me hungry again, less sour about interviewing actors. Besides, how expensive can one tiny baby be?

The worst I can see, out of the corner of one eye, is the terrifying cost of IVF, which seems to go up in increments of fifteen thousand dollars and which, above the age of about forty-two, I once heard described by a doctor as "throwing money into a pit." At thirty-seven, however—which, in what might be the single attractive thing about the fertility industry, I'm learning can be stated as "only thirty-seven"—there is nothing to suggest I need IVF. What I need is IUI, intrauterine insemination, a medicalized version of the turkey baster in which the sperm is launched, via catheter, high up into the womb, minimizing the distance it has to travel to meet the egg. It's cheaper than IVF and much less invasive, requiring in the first instance neither injections nor general anesthetic. That is the good news. The bad news is that for IUI, the broad-stroke success rate for women my age is roughly 12 percent per cycle.

I know this only by accident. One of the things I can never figure out is how, in the face of big life choices, one draws the line between finding out enough to make an informed decision and finding out so much you can't make a decision at all. My approach, so far—except on those occasions when I have failed to shut down a Web site quickly enough—has been denial. From the outset, I decided the only way to proceed without becoming paralyzed by fear was to limit my thinking to a tiny, immediate-term time frame. It's like the thing E. L. Doctorow said in every interview he gave, including to me; that writing a novel was like driving a car down a dark road at night—he couldn't see beyond the arc of the headlights, nonetheless they guided him home. I won't think about money yet, or living arrangements or relationship status. I won't think about the fact I don't have a green card or that my dad lives three thousand miles away. All I need to get home is hope and a measure of ignorance.

The clinic director doesn't mention the 12 percent success rate. To listen to her, you would think no woman over thirty-five has ever had trouble conceiving, and as she talks, I become aware that for my own denial to be sustainable, I must be sure that everyone else in the chain is operating fully in accordance with reality. Patient denial is an act of psychological defense; doctor denial is scalping.

"Here," says the director and hands me a glossy brochure advertising the clinic's special deal—three rounds of IUI for the cost of two, not including drugs, blood tests or unforeseen complications. It's five thousand dollars for the package and if I want, she says, I can pay in installments.

"OK?" she says.

This is not a good moment vis-à-vis my newfound enthusiasm for American health care, but I meekly reply, "Yes." Then I go home and freak out.

How on earth can one buy medical treatment the same way one buys three-for-two cans of beans at Costco? What if, after the second round of IUI, the prognosis looks so grim that any sensible doctor—that is, one not bound by a bulk sales agreement—would recommend a move to IVF? What if I get pregnant on the first round? Doesn't this approach guarantee that, at some level, the doctor's decisions will be based on commercial, not clinical, considerations? If a clinic thinks bulk sales are a good idea, mightn't they think ordering tests I don't need or performing unnecessary procedures are equally good ways to make money?

It reminds me of those dentists who try to push Botox on you while they're flossing your teeth and, sure enough, a day or two later, the hard sell continues with an e-mail not from the doctor but from the clinic manager asking me to "review the financial portion" of my visit and repeating the benefits of buying a "multiple package." Also, she says, because I intend to use donor sperm, I should be aware that the clinic charges three further fees: a $200 handling fee "for all cryopreserved materials," a $100 fee for "thawing the sperm" and a $500 storage fee, should I wish the clinic to hang on to any unused sperm. I send back a polite note saying I have a lot to think about and will be in touch at some point in the future. Two years later, I'm still receiving their newsletter.

"AMAZING," SAYS OLIVER. We are at a French bistro on the corner of Smith Street and Degraw, which is roughly halfway between his apartment and mine. (It's nearer mine, by a whisker. Whenever we have lunch, which we do most weeks, one or other of us checks Google Maps to determine who has the longer walk to the restaurant. Today I have won by about seventy yards.) "What are you going to do?" he says.

"I don't know. I suppose keep looking for a doctor."

It is funny to be here having lunch as we always have, with this discussion about kids on the table. Our lives have both changed since we came to New York—Oliver has written a book and has an American girlfriend; my life is full of L and her baby; we have both acclimated to working at home after ten years in an office—but in some ways, nothing has changed. In spite of a certain surface cynicism, I think we are both still romantic about the country we moved to. Some of my notions about the United States were dispelled within the first few weeks of arriving, but the one that has stubbornly failed to die is that, with the exception of banking technology, America is a place where the future happens first. You can do anything in America. You can change who you are, or at least what you look like, so that seven years after moving, although I am still, at heart, a disheveled English person, I sit across the table from Oliver today with a better haircut, a bigger wardrobe and, after a lot of badgering from L and to the disgust of British friends, shiny white veneers on my teeth. (From a patriotic standpoint, cosmetic dentistry is to British people what burning the flag is to Americans.)

Oliver sits, as he always does, in a dark sweater with a zip up the front, buffer than he was when we lived in Britain and, I notice, with the first gray flecks at his temples. Like many thirtysomething men, he is somewhat mystified by my certainty that I want to have a baby, and can cite a handful of studies testifying to the fact that parents are slightly less happy than people without children.

"A study says . . ." I say, teasingly.

"But I'm genuinely curious. How do you know?"

"I just do. I just know that it's right for me."

What Oliver can see, he says, is that if one *did* want a child, there are advantages to doing it alone, without having to commit to another adult, notionally for life, or figure out the relationship stuff first. Having a baby is one thing; determining whether you're on the same page as your partner about private education or TV during dinner is another order of difficulty entirely. "I can absolutely see the appeal," he says. "Being on your own streamlines about ninety percent of the decisions."

Single men of his age are supposed to feel like this, unsure of "settling down." Single women are not, and every time we talk about it, the same worry yawns open: that all my rationalizations—that what I'm doing is the smart choice, the responsible choice, the choice that untethers having a child from a relationship not built to support it—are a fig leaf for something less admirable. What if, rather than boldly embracing a new kind of family, what I'm doing is standard-issue, male-type commitment phobia? What if, like my weakness for women in gold Rolexes, I am miscasting as feminist victory what is merely the aping of crass male behavior? You'd think that committing to a baby, the most binding commitment of all, would be enough to assuage this fear, but of course that is not what is meant when people talk about commitment phobia. After the birth of L's baby, a couple of youngish guys in her office told her she'd inspired them; what a genius move, they said, to carry on being single while having a baby alone, and they sketched out for her, only half-jokingly, a scenario in which they carried on being single heterosexual guys, going out, getting drunk, dating women, having roommates, but doing the family thing, too. "You know someone has to look after the baby, right?" said L.

I know, of course, that I'm not like those guys. I don't want to party. I don't want to date. I don't even want to go out; I've *been* out. I'm not waiting for something or someone better to come along. Most ludicrously of all, I am not, by some definitions, even single. I call L my "partner," because what else can I say, but that doesn't really cover the ground. Six months after the birth of her baby there is love, and closeness, and reciprocity and occasional hatred that can be triggered only by deep romantic involvement, but the need for separation—not just time apart, but profound, structural circuit breaks between us—is real. It is how our personalities work in combination, the distance on which not just our intimacy but our ability to like and not murder each other depends. As the years go by it becomes increasingly apparent that this is not a relationship phase. We have found our level.

Still, I worry. I hear myself sometimes describing my relationship to others and think I sound like the female half of those heterosexual couples in which the man has persuaded the woman to agree to an open marriage—the tra-la-la, it's-so-wonderful-to-defy-convention breeziness, when you know deep down it's a hideous mess. Not belonging to a well-defined category alarms me. I have no words for what I am to L's baby and I have no idea what she will be to mine and this lack of a language implies something is wrong. And yet whenever I go through these loops, they always end here: with wonder, and amazement, and the most profound gratitude for L's baby and the possibility of my own. There is doubt and anxiety, but the last word is still love.

After lunch, Oliver and I walk west toward Gowanus. We talk about staff changes at work, and the ongoing mystery of American health care. We talk about the cost of fertility treatment. When I told L about the bulk package, I half worried she'd give me the speech about everything in life being negotiable and tell me to go back and ask for a discount. In fact, she took one look at the brochure and said she thought the pricing structure was ludicrous and very obviously a scam. (I have no such worries with Oliver, who is even more English than I am and, to avoid confrontation, prefers to conduct his negotiations in writing, over many months, with someone from customer complaints.)

After bickering for a few moments about who walked the farthest to lunch, we part on the corner of Wyckoff and Bond. "Ah, Brockesy," he says, giving me a hug, "it's been a long, bad-tempered marriage," and although his tone is ironic, the truth of it is that my relationship with L is enabled—subsidized, even—by the nature of my other relationships. Close friendships are supposed to be a crutch of youth, a stopgap until one's other half comes along, but that has not been my experience and it is Oliver, just as much as L, to whom I look to explain my life back to me, just as it's Merope I call to reassure me of the things I already know. "Good one," she says, on the phone from London, when I tell her I am moving on with the baby thing. "Do it, do it, do it."

DR. B'S CLINIC is on the Upper West Side, but not the posh part. (Tenth Avenue, a mile from the park, and way up in the nineties.) There is no water feature in the waiting room or soothing Muzak to move a person to rage. Instead, the TV is tuned to Matt Lauer and his chums, and when the *Today* show ends, the receptionist flips to *TMZ*. It is a month before Christmas and I am ready to commit. I am ready to commit to a fertility doctor.

A word of advice for those shopping in this area in New York; as with high-end gyms in the city, every fertility clinic you encounter, I have discovered, puts out word on the street that "Madonna used it." Poor woman; adoption agencies probably make the same claim. But whereas I can see Madge hanging out at the Equinox gym on Sixty-seventh Street, I have a tough time putting her in this particular waiting room, with its ten-year-old sofas and faded prints of popular artworks on the walls. The clinic is liberal with the insurance it takes, so the waiting room isn't populated with fortysomething suits but with a mixture of ages and races, dressed up and dressed down, so that to my eyes it looks as near to a normal NHS clinic as you are likely to find in Manhattan. Dr. B, a large, bluff man in middle age, fetches me from reception and we walk to his office. No big eyes, no soft voice, merely an adjustment of his tie as he takes a seat behind the desk. "Now," he says. "What can I do for you?"

I explain my situation, rather awkwardly, I suppose, because he says, "OK, so what are you doing for . . ."

"What?"

"You're going to need . . ."

"What?"

He gives me a helpless look. "You know you need sperm, right?"

I burst out laughing. "Yes, I know. I'm choosing a donor."

There will, he explains, be some exploratory tests and then, all going well, we will try a cycle of IUI with no drugs. He says this with a shrug, as if to say maybe it'll work, maybe it won't, then pulls out a chart from his desk drawer, correlating historical birth rates with the age of the mother. There is a big spike at the end, accounting for modern women having babies later and later and which, he says, "evolution hasn't caught up with yet." He smiles broadly. "But let's see what we can do!"

For the next ten minutes, we chat about other things: my job, the state of the world, our tastes in TV, books and movies. The conversation flows naturally, but it also feels like a discreet but formal phase of the interview designed to ensure that I find him simpatico. And I do. I like him, right up to the point when he learns I work for the *Guardian* and gets very animated about Julian Assange.

Something has happened to the *Guardian* since I moved to New York. When I arrived, it was an office of four people in a building in Midtown, with a communal bathroom down the hall and a children's talent agency next door, so that every morning the elevator was full of Baby Junes doing high kicks. No one would return my calls, and if they did, by some miracle, they would invariably start the conversation with "Is that the *Manchester Guardian*?"

"It was called that fifty years ago, now it's just the *Guardian*."

After a long pause: "I'm sorry, I don't deal with foreign press."

All that changed after WikiLeaks. Now it's a loft in SoHo, one hundred people strong, and New York is crawling with former colleagues from London. There are so many of them in my neighborhood, a section of the deli on the corner has been opened up to British confectionary (Curly Wurlys, Aeros, a few dusty Lion bars). Oliver and I grumble about this—what was the point of moving when the entire office moved with us?—but it is of course deeply gratifying and I take as much passive credit for WikiLeaks and, later, Edward Snowden as I can, although I had as much to do with them as Cindy Adams did with Watergate.

Dr. B gives a short, rousing speech in praise of Julian Assange, whom he depicts as a folk hero ill served by the media generally and my newspaper in particular.

"He's kind of a weirdo," I say.

"Of course he is! No one else would take on interests that powerful." Then he itemizes all the things big government isn't telling us.

"I can't tell if you're on the right or the left."

Dr. B looks indignant. "Neither. I don't believe in those categories."

"Oh, god, you're not a Libertarian, are you?"

He smiles and raises his eyebrows, which I take to be an invitation not to take him too seriously. "I describe myself as an anarcho-capitalist."

We don't get around to money until the very end of the interview. It is nine hundred dollars per insemination, plus the cost of drugs, blood tests and ultrasounds, and I will pay only for what I need. Without insurance coverage, says Dr. B, it can get expensive very quickly and he will work with me to keep the costs down. Perhaps this is a sales pitch, too, but it works. Instinctively, I trust him.

Then he says something that shocks me. "Do you believe in god?"

I am so taken aback I laugh. "No. I mean, no. Not for the purposes of this conversation."

"I assumed you wouldn't." He looks embarrassed. "But I have to ask, because if you do, there are parts of this process you might find . . . problematic."

"Don't worry. I don't think you're assisting me in going to hell."

"OK!" He gets up, skirts the desk and, showing me to the door, offers a hand to shake. "Very good, very nice to meet you and I'll see you next week."

The second I get outside, I call Oliver. "Would you let someone who thinks Julian Assange is a hero rummage around in your ovaries?" I ask.

"Um," says Oliver. "I mean, the two things aren't really related, are they?"

"No. Although there's a broad question of judgment."

"Did you like him apart from that?"

"Oh, I'm not sure I disliked him for it. If anything, I liked him more for the fact he's not an establishment drone."

"I wouldn't worry about it, then."

"I mean, he's wrong about Assange, but . . ."

"Yeah. As long as he knows what he's doing with your . . ."

"Yeah. Right. OK. Good."

ONE OF THE THINGS you have to get used to when you are a British person embarking on fertility treatment in the United States is the pace of it all. In a small country like Britain, the law of supply and demand is such that there are more women wanting donor sperm than there are donors to give it, so that even in the private clinics there's often a waiting list. In America, where no one with adequate resources waits for anything, you have a chat with your doctor, schedule a date, call the donor bank, which bikes the sperm round to the clinic, and off you go. You might have spent six months or six years deciding to do this; but you could, potentially, be pregnant within a month of first seeing your doctor.

I do not anticipate this will happen to me—getting pregnant without a struggle still seems too outlandish, too decisively *female,* to fit the rest of my life. But the very fact that it might, or that it might be revealed to be conclusively impossible, makes the week before the last diagnostic test feel like the pause at the top of a roller coaster. If I want to avoid the possibility of total destruction, now is the time to get out. As of this moment, I'm a thirty-eight-year-old woman who wants but doesn't have children, a sad state but that's life, what can you do, maybe next year. If I let this go further, through diagnostic testing and beyond, I will potentially be a thirty-eight-, thirty-nine-, forty-plus-year-old woman who is trying and failing to have children, which sounds to me like a different order of upset altogether. It's not just the fear that the treatment might fail. It's the fear that it might fail over months and years and still end in nothing. It's the fear that my standard damage limitation response— "maybe I wasn't that bothered in the first place"—will be impossible to pull off. If Dr. B discovers something catastrophic when he examines my fallopian tubes next week, a whole new schedule of adjustment begins. I will have to grieve for the biological child I can't have and reconfigure what my next decade might look like. I will have to deal with my animosity toward people with children. There will be the sheer bloody hassle of having to accommodate new facts about myself, at an age when I'm inclined to think I have it somewhat worked out. Ovaries that don't work shouldn't impact a woman's fundamental identity, but I have a feeling they do, so that the choice, at this stage, seems to be between two negative self-images: that of a woman trying and failing to conceive and that of a woman too scared even to try.

And then there is L. I can't begin to guess how infertility might affect our relationship. But given my bottomless capacity for resentment, I assume it won't be for the better. Suddenly, I understand why women my age who want children nonetheless let the years slide by. Better to wake up one day and, without having made an active decision, realize it is over and the option to conceive has expired. In this scenario, it's not that you "couldn't have children" but that you "didn't have children," a presentation of the facts relieved of its diagnostic burden. The self-help industry assures us it's always better to try and fail than to not try at all, but in the case of women's fertility, there is a strong rationale for avoiding "failure" at all costs, given the way in which that failure is perceived.

For the rest of the week, I distract myself with business as usual. I meet Oliver for lunch (a Vietnamese sandwich shop in Park Slope, a decisive win on his part). I research a piece about people who die unexpectedly on airplanes, tracking down a Swedish woman who tells me what it was like to sit next to a corpse for nine hours on a full flight from Sweden to Kenya. On the weekend, I go to Costco with L and the baby. As we cruise the overlit aisles, trying samples and reliving our greatest Costco hits—this was where we bought the crab paste that got recalled; here, the site of our most legendary impulse purchase, a machine that vacuum packs meat—I try to imagine another child in the cart, this one with my face on it. Will we look like a family? I wonder. Or like two disparate people and some babies who've teamed up to buy bulk?

I am not supposed to shrink from describing what happens next. I should be proud to reclaim the language of female anatomy. Unfortunately, while it strikes me that "testicle" can raise a titter and "penis" can be kind of fun, and that post–Eve Ensler even "vagina" is less burdensome than it was, once you get into the realm of hard-core female reproductive machinery—FALLOPIAN, OVARY, CERVIX, UTERUS—I find it very hard not to feel that I'm letting the side down. Womb. Glands. Tubes. Eggs. If I could write about my experiences while avoiding these words, I would. In the event, all I can do is apologize to anyone who finds this kind of thing as distasteful as I do and recommend skipping ahead to chapter 8, where there is blood, yes, but also some lovely Vancouver scenery and a walk-on appearance by Al Gore.

For those still with me: here is Dr. B, at the foot of the gurney, firing a tiny jet from a water cannon around my fallopian tubes while following its progress on the ultrasound. "Look," he says, pointing at the screen, a black expanse streaked with silver. It looks like a shit version of Space Invaders.

"Hmmm," I say, as if we were standing before a painting in a gallery. We wait. And wait.

"I'm not seeing any movement through the fallopian tubes," says Dr. B. "Hang on." He adjusts the tube and points to the screen. "See? This is where the water is going in and . . . nothing is coming out the other end."

I frown as if making intelligent sense of this, although the truth is medical details hit my brain like street directions; if I'm lucky, I can grab hold of a single orientating term to feed into the Internet afterward. Otherwise, I go on the mood of the room. This one isn't good.

The absorption of bad news can be forestalled by the more pressing task of dealing with the feelings of the person who's giving it. For about twenty seconds after we got my mother's terminal cancer diagnosis, she and I looked at the mustachioed oncologist and thought, my god, this poor man is in agony. One imagines that a death sentence will unleash violent emotions, or perhaps paralysis. What one doesn't anticipate is the embarrassment. As Dr. B stares at the screen, I feel the weight of his discomfort more keenly than the findings.

"No," he says eventually, looking a little cross. "Nothing's coming through the other end. OK, we have a problem." I get dressed and, after a short wait, adjourn to his office, where he prints out a screenshot of my fallopian tubes and places it on the desk between us. It looks like grainy satellite imagery of enemy ground the U.S. Air Force is preparing to bomb.

"OK, there are some options," says Dr. B. The hydrosonogram is not a foolproof procedure and sometimes produces false negatives.

Maybe nothing is wrong and we should start the treatment regardless. On the other hand, he says, maybe the test is right and I have blocked fallopian tubes, in which case there's no way I'll get pregnant without intervention—at the very least, an operation called a hysteroscopy, in which a tiny endoscopic camera will be threaded into my uterus, so the doctor can identify the problem and potentially fix it. It could be fibroids, it could be nothing, it could be something. My call. I am, after all, the paying customer.

I wish I could say that after this consultation, I suspend my moratorium on research and self-educate to Ph.D. standard, like Nick Nolte in *Lorenzo's Oil*. At the very least, I should be feverishly Googling "hysteroscopy" and its related terms. But every time I think about researching the operation, I am overcome with inertia and something else, a primitive sense that by focusing on the bad things I will increase the chances of them happening. The most I can bring myself to do is to Google "blocked fallopian tubes," a search that brings up a lot of testimony from desperately unhappy women at the tail end of multiyear fights to get pregnant. Blocked tubes, I read, account for some 20 percent of infertility.

And yet I'm reluctant to go in for elective surgery. The operation, said Dr. B, can be conducted only under general anesthetic and taking even the tiny risks associated with that seems obscene. My mind ranges back to the chemo unit. Bravery in the face of cancer is admirable; bravery in the face of an avoidable operation feels like a parody of those with real problems.

I do something then that is more emotional than practical: I look to see how doctors would be handling my situation if I still lived in Britain. If the hysteroscopy is considered all right at home, under a health-care system so strapped for cash that most NHS managers would rather die than green-light an "unnecessary procedure," then I tell myself I have nothing to worry about. If the Brits don't go for it, then neither will I.

It takes two minutes at my computer to find what I'm looking for: guidelines issued to doctors by the Royal College of Obstetricians and Gynaecologists. Just reading those words soothes me. Here we go, the royal standard, the firm hand of authority from a world-class health system that doesn't ask you, the least qualified person in the room, to make clinical decisions, but instead tells you what's good for you and you can either like it or move to America.

The advice laid down to British doctors by the RCOG is that the hysteroscopy is a "successful, safe and well-tolerated" operation, albeit one associated with "significant pain, anxiety and embarrassment" on the part of the woman. In spite of that last bit, the governing body recommends that doctors conduct it under local anesthetic, because, to paraphrase, buck up ladies, that's life. (One wonders if it was a man or a woman who wrote these guidelines.) It is hard not to laugh at this, the difference in the two cultures' ideas of pain management. In Britain, whether it hurts or not, it is assumed you will take it on the chin and be grateful that anyone bothered with you in the first place. Years before moving to America, I'd gone for minor eye surgery at Moorfields in London, and when I inquired, timorously, of the consultant, "Is it going to hurt?" he gave me a flat yes and a spiky look just for asking.

In America, by contrast, any degree of pain, like any degree of heat or cold in a poorly temperature-controlled house, is considered less a fact of life than a failure on the part of the service provider. In my biased view, this makes pain as a concept harder to control, although this is, I understand, as much a hangover from my mother's parenting as a function of cultural difference. In the chemo unit, at home with her back pain, throughout her entire life, it was my mother's core belief that something will hurt in proportion to the fuss that one makes about it. As a result, in very limited circumstances—blood tests, immunizations, minor operations—I can enjoy pain; it makes me feel important. My eye operation hurt like hell, but it gave me something to kick against and allowed me to congratulate myself for being my mother's brave little soldier.

After reading the RCOG guidelines I decide I'll have the operation. But bristling with my mother's machismo and something like patriotic pride, I call the clinic to request it under local anesthetic. Twenty minutes later the nurse calls back and says under no circumstances will Dr. B operate without a general anesthetic and doubts any doctor in Manhattan will; it is simply too painful.

Something occurs to me then. If I had been with a male partner trying to conceive the regular way, I would in all likelihood have been trying and failing to get pregnant for months or even years by now, my two blocked tubes undiagnosed and untreated. I would, potentially, already have become That Woman, whose inability to conceive overshadows every other aspect of her life. By doing it the artificial way, I have shrunk the agony down to less than a week. Fear gives way to relief and then to euphoria. A third self-image presents itself: I am immensely lucky! This is all for the best! Thank god I'm half single, half in a same-sex relationship and not in a conventional marriage! Four days later, I go in for the procedure.

L has a meeting that morning and offers to cancel and come with me, but it gives me a small sense of victory to renounce my own needs and so I turn her down, then get the added buzz of resenting her for not overriding me. (She knows I am doing this, and won't override me partly in retaliation for not stating my needs plainly. I tell myself this is completely unjust given that we can't change our natures and there's a minuscule chance I might DIE here.) Oliver, with whom I do not play these games, travels up from Park Slope for an eight a.m. start and sits with me in the prep room, where he spends thirty minutes trying to get Wi-Fi and communicate to the anesthetist that he isn't my husband—unsuccessfully on both counts. Just before I'm wheeled in, my phone buzzes; it's L, texting me a photo from the summer of me holding the baby in an orchard. We are both smiling at the camera. I send her back kisses.

When I wake up, Oliver is at my bedside. "You're not making any sense," he says.

"Huh?"

"You're talking an amazing amount of shit."

I still occasionally worry about this. Given that I emigrated on the strength of the drugs for three fillings, I can't imagine what unfiltered junk flew out from my subconscious after being out cold. With Oliver's help, I get off the gurney and, after retreating behind a screen to get dressed and thanking the anesthetist—"Good luck to you both," he says, and we blush—we make our way upstairs to reception. Depending on what Dr. B found down those tunnels—space debris? Scar tissue? Cobwebs?—it is possible I am about to hit the end of the road, in which case, I decide, I will simply push it to the back of my mind along with all the other things I put off indefinitely, like figuring out what I think about life after death and finding an alternative to Time Warner Cable. Eventually, I have to believe, I'll come to terms with it.

Dr. B appears and beckons me to follow him into his office.

"A buildup of matter," he says genially. "Quite normal, very common and I've cleared both tubes out."

"What kind of matter? What's it made of?" He says some words I don't catch—some sort of tissue, possibly beginning with *F*. Anyway, "Water is flowing in both directions," he says. "We're good to go."

This is great news. There are no further preliminaries. I gulp; now I will actually have to go through with it.

FIVE

Sperm

MY GRANDFATHER on my mother's side was a convicted murderer and child molester who abused all eight of his children. He was an alcoholic, a drug addict and almost certainly a psychopath, and was released after serving six years in prison for murder—of an old man during a robbery—two years before my mother was born. Most of us understand intuitively that the sins of the father don't transfer down the generations in any measurable way, but I understand this more keenly than most. This man, my mother's father, killed, robbed, cheated, beat his wife, raped his children and went on mad rampages with an ax, before keeling over from a brain hemorrhage brought on by the substance abuse that runs rampant in the family. And yet my mother was good, kind, just and loving, funny, cheerful and sane.

A few weeks after my dinner with William in London, he sent me a long, thoughtful e-mail telling me he had taken my request very seriously, calling his mother in Spain and discussing it at length, before coming to the conclusion that it would simply be too hard for him to father a child and not be involved in its life. To my surprise I was overwhelmed by relief. William supported what I was doing and wished me all the love and luck in the world and I was very touched by this, by both the lengths he had gone to and the concern of his e-mail. Now, with the clear conscience of having explored some alternatives, I was free to do as I pleased.

This is a tricky part of the story for me. Characterizing my relationship with L is hard, but in some ways characterizing the donor process is harder. It is the place where, in casual conversation with others, I'm most likely to feel curiosity lean toward prurient interest, where I find the question of navigating the line between being transparent and being gross the most difficult to call. There may come a day when it is as regular as milk to share details of one's sperm donor—when there is a language less alienating to describe it than this, and that feels less compromising of one's child's essential privacy. But we are not there yet, and as I begin searching, I realize I have no idea how to calibrate this choice. Is it the biggest of my life, or one that is essentially meaningless? Underplay the donor and you risk turning the guy into the elephant in the room; go on about him too much and you risk pathologizing your child's background. No matter how often I tell myself it doesn't work like this, the fear of doing it wrong—of making the wrong decisions, with generation-deep consequences—is there from the outset.

At my desk, scrolling through profiles, I look for characteristics that align with my own. I want someone clever, which in this context means educated. I want someone with dark hair. I want someone whose favorite film isn't *Once Upon a Time in America* or *Titanic*. In the absence of a metric for gauging a man's humor or internal beauty or moral worth, I want someone tall and basically symmetrical. A choice is superficial only if it is made at the expense of deeper considerations and so, although I reject sperm donors on criteria that would outrage me if applied in real life by men, to women, I tell myself I'm not doing anything wrong. I want someone with a background similar to my own, to minimize the possibility of my child glamorizing the donor and also to lessen the number of items on my to-do list—take her to Peru; teach her Mandarin—to fill in the missing parts of her identity. This means a white, Anglo-Saxon (or, at a pinch, Catholic) American with western European origins, educated to the same or higher standard that I was—but not a writer, because I know writers and they're messed up and I don't want a journalist, either, in case I know him, or he's a bad one and I dilute my good journalist's genes with shoddy ones. I want someone with talents different from my own but that I think of as equally interesting (but not too interesting), i.e., not a marketing executive or a mime artist.

It strikes me that neither L, nor most of my male friends, nor I myself, in fact, would clear these filters, L on the basis of her job and religion, my male friends, who are funny and intelligent and most of whom can't throw a ball, for reasons of height or athletic ability. And when I look at my own genetic heritage I can only laugh. If there is a single scenario in which having a murderer and a pedophile in the family tree is an advantage, it is here, now, as I sit at my desk trying to parse donor profiles for signs of degeneracy. Imagine the profile if I was an egg donor: five foot eight, 135 pounds, good liberal arts education and two generations out from your worst nightmare.

As for the narrowness of my selection criteria, all I can think is that it's a mistake to see this exercise as equivalent to friendship or dating. I keep reading magazine pieces about "sperm donor parties," or "egg-freezing parties," as if having a child this way were not a series of sober, unnerving decisions but some mad version of a hen party. The donor banks are just as bad. They're all called things like "Infertility Solutions," making them sound as if they have a sideline in targeted killings, but when you visit the Web sites, most are set up to look like quasi dating services, their grammar and architecture reinforcing the lie that you are choosing a husband, a coparent and the progenitor of exactly 50 percent of your child's face and personality. They go to great lengths to avoid the word "catalog," but that's what it is, pages of donor profiles with vital statistics, photos and numbers attached. Some of the Web sites even have a little shopping basket icon in the right-hand corner of the home page and an option to "check out"—both entirely for show, given that you can't do any of this without making at least one phone call. Still, in the early stages of the search, you might be forgiven for thinking you were browsing online for a bath mat at Target.

Everything is extra. Thirty-five dollars for the guy's baby photos. (Guidelines vary from state to state, but in New York, you can see only photos of the donor as a child.) Fifty dollars for an audio file. Some donor banks offer a "silhouette" of the donor as an adult, which would be hilarious if it wasn't so creepy. What next—his breath in a jar to rule out halitosis? Handwritten personal profiles that delineate tastes, preferences and motivations for donating cost extra, too, although "impressions from the desk staff" are free of charge and also free of content. For example, "attractive, with a friendly manner" and "seemed quiet, but kind," assessments it is impossible not to scrutinize as code.

It feels, simultaneously, like a deeply personal choice and like a parody of choice, one in which each further detail only adds to the sense of how shallow the data pool. And yet it is almost impossible not to invest it with meaning.

"You know," says Oliver over a beer one night, "there's a philosophical argument to be made for blind sperm allocation, where you can't find out anything at all."

He is needling me and it works. "Genes matter," I say fiercely, then realize I don't know to what extent I believe this. Sperm banks trade on the bogus idea that if you buy enough extras, you can filter your way to the ideal child—a claim, by the way, with a guaranteed 100 percent success rate, given that once a woman is pregnant, she is inclined to consider her baby not only ideal but inevitable. So I see the logic of "random selection." It states, quite clearly, that we have no control over the genetic makeup of the child we produce; that all we can do is act in love and blind faith and hope for the best.

Still, I resist the idea of blind allocation. It seems monstrously impertinent, seeming to hold me and other women in my position to higher existential standards—that is, standards governed by rationalism rather than the gloopy emotional swamp out of which most of our motivations emerge—than women having kids with a husband's sperm. The choice of donor may be meaningless in terms of a controllable outcome, but there is still huge emotional value to be had from making it.

HOW, THEN, to make the choice? For a single afternoon, I wonder if cost should be one of the factors.

There are, it turns out, as in every other consumer goods sector, cheap sperm banks and expensive sperm banks. The cheap ones have chaotic Web sites and no apparent door policy in terms of who can donate—the equivalent of Match.com but for sperm—where the cost is a couple of hundred dollars cheaper than the average and no one edits the profiles. I see one in which the donor, an unemployed twenty-two-year-old, answers the question "Why do you want to be a sperm donor?" with the answer "Need the money," and wonder if this is the most honest man I will find.

Out of curiosity one day, I click on the catalog of egg donors and it is then that I notice a startling disparity. Brains come from the dad and looks from the mum, right? And so, while male donors at the expensive banks are almost all educated to at least the level of a master's degree, female egg donors of equivalent value are by and large indifferently educated. They have high school diplomas and degrees in sports science. But they all to a woman look like Ukrainian models.

"You know it's probably all Dr. B's, right?" says L.

"That's gross."

"Think about it. I bet every kid conceived in this place comes from his sperm."

Variations on this theme become a running joke. "For all I know, it could be the janitor's!" I say to friends and it raises a laugh, as if this were the most hilariously terrible fate that could befall an educated woman—*janitor's sperm*! Imagine! Then we sober up and acknowledge that, of course, there is nothing wrong with being a janitor and the act of choosing a sperm donor sadly flushes out the fascist in all of us. It formalizes the worst aspects of human nature. It makes us mean. It turns us all into John Galliano. Legitimize these impulses and before you know it we will be trading babies on eBay, classified by height, weight, IQ and color, for anyone to buy and return.

This is ostensibly what the legislation is for; to save us from ourselves and prevent the advent of "designer" babies. In reality, of course, a lot of the legislation around fertility treatment is based on religious principles designed not to rule out eugenics but to prevent the "wrong" kind of people from having children. In Italy, use of sperm or egg donors was banned across the board until the high court overturned the law in early 2014, but the right to assisted reproduction is still restricted for "single parents, same-sex couples and women beyond childbearing age." An estimated four thousand Italians a year go abroad seeking help, mostly to Spain.

In Switzerland, donor sperm can be used only by heterosexual married couples who have been married for at least a year before treatment. (It's a shame they don't transfer some of this moral zeal to their banking laws.)

The UK has among the most progressive laws in Europe. There are no restrictions on who can be treated, but to prevent accidental inbreeding, there are limitations on the number of families to which an individual donor can contribute; in this case, ten. In Norway it's eight, in Sweden it's six. In New Zealand, it is a maximum of ten kids among a maximum of four families. In France, there are no restrictions on sibling numbers within a single (heterosexual) family, but no more than six families may be helped by a single donor.

And then there is America. Guidelines issued by the American Society for Reproductive Medicine recommend that each donor be limited to no more than twenty-five births per 850,000 of population and most responsible sperm banks impose narrower restrictions than this. But in terms of actual inviolable laws, there are none. There is no central tracking system for children born of sperm or egg donors and no legal obligation for the clinics to submit records. It is completely and utterly unregulated.

Officially, I am appalled by this. It must, I think, encourage a cow-

boy mind-set among fertility doctors. Secretly, however, as with my entire push-me, pull-me relationship with American health care, I am
delighted by the freedoms of the American system; the lack of moral
judgment it implies and the amount of information I can find out about
the donor. And while I watch as friends in Britain struggle to source
sperm, I have access to more than I know what to do with. (Since the
laws changed in 2005, sperm donors in the UK have had to forfeit their
anonymity, so that children can get in touch with them when they turn
eighteen. As a result, the number of donors has dropped, while the
number of women seeking to use them has risen. I have friends back
home who report applying to a donor bank for sperm only to discover
there are only a handful of donors on the list—and far fewer identifying
details than one is provided with in the United States. If you want to
know how tall the donor's siblings are or what they do for a living,
tough. If you want Jewish sperm, tough, there's a shortage and the sperm
bank might not even make that information available, because, by some
skewed logic, it is thought to constitute "religious discrimination." And
by the way, you can't import it from Israel—a friend in London tried
and was told the regulatory body in Britain doesn't allow sperm into the
country that doesn't meet the country's strict compliancy laws. "Can't I
just take it on the plane in a freezer bag?" she said to the doctor in Tel
Aviv. He might've done it, too, she said, if he hadn't known she was a
journalist and suspected a setup. "I suppose technically it's people traf-
ficking.")

"He looks spectrumy," I say to L on the phone one day. It is the middle of the working week and I am supposed to be writing about the war
against Christmas. Instead, I am picking holes in a photo of a five-year-
old boy.

"He's cute!" she says, looking at the screen in her office.

"Is he?" I glance down the profile and see that he has grown up to be a twenty-nine-year-old computer analyst. "Do you think that means Bill Gates or the IT guy?"

"What does the rest of the profile say?"

Farther down the page, the desk clerk describes him as "shy," evidently code for weird, even though I am shy myself and, with the exception of L, can't tolerate extroverts. I look at him again. He is squinting slightly, looking anxiously at the camera, and it's at that point that I feel a strange shift in perspective. As I consider this nerdy little guy in his disastrous sweater and massive glasses, I have a surge of maternal feeling. I don't want his sperm, but if he were mine, I would kill anyone for critiquing him as I had.

"I don't really approve," says Gavin. It's Friday night and we are drinking martinis at the Oyster Bar in Grand Central station. The place was empty an hour ago. Now it's thronged with men in suits, ties loosened, lunging toward the bar. (I'm supposed to be cutting down on drinking, but I figure one can't hurt. After all, I'm only thirty-eight.)

"How can you not approve, you're a gay man!"

"What does that have to do with it?" Every time I talk with Gavin about this he rotates between supportive and sucked-lemon face. My joke about janitor's sperm hasn't landed well and right now he is going the full sucked lemon.

"It sounds like eugenics," he says.

"What? So I should go for the ugly stupid guys, just to be fair?"

"But it's so superficial."

"Everything's superficial! I don't see you picking out the monsters on Grindr."

"But you don't give someone a chance to show you their charm."

"But it's not a relationship!"

"Yes. But."

"What?"

"Well . . ."

"What?"

"I wouldn't get picked in this kind of selection." Ah.

"That's ridiculous. You have a really good degree. You have a great job in journalism. You're really attractive."

"I'm too old."

"You're only forty!"

He looks depressed. "You know that in gay years that's about seventy-five."

"I would totally take your sperm if I thought you'd give it to me."

"Really?"

"Of course."

Gavin cheers up and we order another round. "That's the nicest thing you've ever said to me."

He is right, of course. It does sound awful, all of it, right down to "using" a sperm donor. The language is cold and commercial and it makes men feel bad, as if the criteria on which my choice of donor is based were a referendum on them personally. I suspect there's an aesthetic dimension, too. Liberals are supposed to applaud a woman's right to choose, whether that be to abort, to have a baby and walk away from her spouse, or to be abandoned and still raise her children with dignity, so that right-wing initiaves encouraging women to marry are mocked by people like me as hopelessly confused. But I know plenty of lefties who cringe at the idea of relatively wealthy women having children alone via sperm donor, either because, when they try to imagine their own lives minus their beloved fathers, it makes them feel sad, or because it seems like yet another example of privileged people gaming the system.

"But why shouldn't I have one if I want one?" I say to Gavin, who doesn't believe that having a child is an inalienable right.

"Yes, and I want a five-bedroom house in Chelsea, Emma. But we can't all get what we want, can we."

WITH THE HYSTEROSCOPY behind me, Dr. B schedules my first round of IUI for the end of December. In anticipation, I am supposed to cut out alcohol entirely, but there are Christmas parties to attend and I tell myself champagne doesn't count. At one of them, someone sidles up to me, ostensibly to rescue me from a man explaining game theory to me, but really to find out where I am in my process. He's a good-ish friend I don't see all that often and I do the mental math to figure out how he knows. Rats. I always tell one person too many and that person is always a blabbermouth.

"You're not—are you?" he says.

"No!" I hold up the champagne.

"But you're trying?"

"About to start."

I don't particularly mind his questioning. His own domestic situation is complicated, so the conversation is more or less balanced. More generally, however, I'm still having a tough time figuring out how to talk about this. It seems to me almost impossible to give an honest account of myself that is neither too defensive, too jolly nor too grossly revealing, so that I spend a lot of that season wandering around feeling actively aphasic.

I keep thinking about my mother. She believed in genes, rather perversely. Ignoring her father, she put her sanity down to the genes she inherited from her sainted mother, a woman who died at the age of twenty-one, when my mother was two, and of whom she had absolutely no memory. My mother was adamant that it was thanks to this woman that she escaped the hell of her father's personality. "Strong women, strong genes," she would say to me, indicating her maternal forebears, and I think about this a lot at my desk while I'm scrolling through profiles. Perhaps there is a genetic basis for resilience and renewal. But I tend to think my mother's ability to break the cycle, to move away from South Africa and marry a man like my dad while some of her sisters married men like their father, was less a question of genetic programming than shrewd decision making. (Of course, there is an argument that the ability to make a shrewd decision is itself genetically encoded, but I don't have the bandwidth to wrestle with that.) More than that, it was a question of vision. My mother understood that when you're in a tight spot, the illusion of agency can be almost as powerful as the real thing. She couldn't change her background but she could choose "strong women, strong genes." She could choose to interpret her genetic inheritance as matrilineal. Above all, she could choose an idea of herself as the author of her own fortune.

It is almost impossible for someone of my generation living in New York not to believe that therapy would have been good for my mother, but in its absence, she made the smartest choice of all: to recast her silence about what happened to her in childhood not as repression or denial or any of the words we use for survivors of child sex abuse who haven't "dealt with" their experiences, but rather, as a gift. My childhood was unblighted by what had happened to her and it was only much later that I understood what she had done, a remarkable act, not just for me perhaps, but for her, too. The power to withhold has, historically, been the only one available to women but it is no less profound for that, and for my mother it was the beginning of happiness. Her life after leaving South Africa was an act of will, but more than that it was an act of imagination, an ability—a talent, really—to look beyond the experience of her background and see other possibilities.

I DON'T LISTEN to the audio files. I don't try to find the guy, even though there is so much information it would probably take me less than a day. I draw what feels like a sensible line between finding out enough and trying to find out too much. This is not gene selection; it is the selection of the story of how my child came to be and, through a combination of vital statistics, familiarity of background, a subtle but readable implication that he is a Democrat, and his use of the word "tremendous," which signals to me a certain wryness and enthusiasm, I make my choice. In other words, on nothing substantive at all. What matters is it's my choice and I make it.

I pay extra for ID disclosure, enabling any child I produce to trace the donor when she turns eighteen. I decide how much to buy—enough for three cycles—then fill in a form with my credit card details and return it to the donor bank, along with payment for almost $2,000: that is, $500 per vial plus $150 to courier it in a freezer bag across town to the clinic. When I call to confirm my request, I half expect the receptionist to laugh and tell me this whole process is a prank and what on earth am I doing, trying to buy genetic material over the phone as if it were the lunch special at Zabar's? Instead, after I mumble out "need to order some sperm," she puts me through to the lab, where a technician will check to see if what I want is available.

"Number?" says the man.

I give him the donor number. There is a clacking of keys, followed by a short pause. Then, with the smoothness of a sommelier fielding a wine order at dinner, he says, "An excellent choice."

SIX

January
2014

A MONTH AFTER the operation I'm in Dr. B's office, snow jacket limp on the back of my chair. Outside, large-scale things are happening. Russian tanks are threatening Crimea. Greece is bankrupt and thinking of leaving the EU. Edward Snowden is in Hong Kong, scattering national secrets and the Scots are deliberating on whether to secede. In here, however, there is only one headline and that is that after weeks of monitering, my eggs are ready. This is it, says Dr. B. I can come in tomorrow and, after waiting for an hour for the sperm to defrost, finally get this show on the road.

"Oh," he says, seeing me to the door. "One other thing." And he asks if I'd like L to be present when the insemination takes place. He shrugs. "Some people find it nice to involve their partners."

For the last few weeks, everything at the clinic has been blissfully dull. Fertility treatment is repetitive. You sit in the same reception area week after week, waiting for your name to be called. You go to the blood room, roll up your sleeve, offer your arm, make conversation with the nurse, go in for the ultrasound, make conversation with the nurse, go back to the waiting room, wait to be called by the doctor and finally go in to discuss the prognosis. In between these engagements, you watch TV in the waiting room and listen to the receptionist as she shouts, "YOU GOT YOUR PERIOD? OK, COME IN TOMORROW" down the phone, roughly once every six minutes. It takes me an embarrassingly long while to realize that each time this happens, another poor woman's hopes have been dashed for that month.

The point of all this activity is to ascertain, to within a twelve-hour period and by measuring estrogen levels in the blood and follicle size via ultrasound, when ovulation is about to occur. I hadn't even known, prior to this, that a woman is fertile only for a handful of days every month, nor that sperm can live in the body for up to five days. Now there is no corner of my fertility, no fluctuation in my blood, that can slink past the doctors unmeasured. There is still an element of guesswork; it is possible for the doctors to overshoot and miss ovulation, which doesn't preclude a pregnancy, but is seen as a professional misfire. Otherwise, everything builds toward that perfect point in the month, the day before ovulation and the patient's most fertile window: Insemination Day!

First, however, I must survive this moment with Dr. B at the door. Being tied to a schedule this month has been such a relief that I forgot there are still things to decide. The thing is, says Dr. B, that fertility treatment, particularly when there's a donor element, can be hard and excluding, and involving the patient's partner in the treatment room, even to the extent of inviting him or her to operate the syringe full of sperm, can give that person a feeling of inclusion. I feel myself blush. Clearly, he's in favor of L's being present, either because it gives him a warm, fuzzy feeling or to neutralize some latent ambivalence he has about helping to create single mothers. I try to imagine the scene: me, stressed out and half naked on a gurney; L, holding the catheter and rolling her eyes; the medical staff, milling around trying not to intrude on our beautiful moment. I don't think I want her there—I don't want anyone there; it's embarrassing—but when I imagine asking L if she wants to be involved, I realize I don't want to give her an opportunity to say no, either.

"Er, no, thanks," I say.

"OK," says Dr. B, maintaining eye contact for half a second too long. "As you like."

In different circumstances, perhaps I would go in for the whole honey-you-detonate-the-plunger thing. Clearly it makes the doctors feel good and is helpful to some couples. And symbolism matters. The baby is learning to talk at the moment and he calls me Emma, or Amma, or sometimes, through early name confusion, Mamma, which makes L cross, a response I think of as ungenerous until years later, when one of my daughters goes through the same phase, and when she calls L Mummy I can't stand it—can't STAND it—at which point I have to laugh and acknowledge we have both been absurd. But these signifiers matter. They shape how we see things, how we decide where one of us ends and the other begins, and on that basis alone, having L involved in the insemination seems wrong. We are not doing this together. She is not my coparent. The symbolism needs to reflect that.

There is a cold, mean streak in me that thinks trying to involve the partner in the treatment room is ludicrous under any circumstances. Surely there's a dignity in allowing things to be what they are? In recognizing that even if the doctors hand out cigarettes after the insemination, this is and always will be a medical procedure that involves only one half of the couple. Pretending otherwise—grafting on a parody of the "normal" way of doing things—risks making the treatment seem sadder, just as choosing a sperm donor will continue to feel sad, or bad, or weird, as long as it's tied to conventions associated with choosing a spouse.

"Hello, hello!" says Dr. B, breezing in. It is a week before Christmas and he is full of good cheer.

"Hello!" I reply brightly.

"So! What's going on? What's the gossip? What's the news about Edward Snowden?"

"I could tell you, but I'd have to kill you," I say weakly. While Dr. B moves around the room, assembling utensils for the insemination, we talk about Russia, and Greece, and then Scotland comes up and I stop blandly going along with his views. "It would be lunacy if they left," I say.

"Not at all!" he says, holding up the vial of sperm, for me to check the details on the label. "They have the oil money, why shouldn't they want independence?" He asks me what I think about Ukrainian sovereignty and I try and fail to summon an opinion.

"There'll be another war," says Dr. B darkly.

"Right."

"Seriously. Figure out a strategy, because it's coming."

"What's your strategy?"

"Ah. My strategy—my philosophy for living—is the three Gs." He loads the syringe with a substance that is, gram for gram, more expensive than the world's finest heroin, although less expensive, perhaps, than marrying someone you're not into in order to have a baby—to shoot up through the catheter, to the cervix and beyond.

"What are the three Gs?"

Dr. B looks sideways at the nurse, who is absorbed in a task at the desk. "I'll tell you another time," he says and lowers his head. I look up at the white-paneled ceiling.

Doctors, like most creative professionals, have their own distinct styles and for his part Dr. B doesn't favor the use of any particular catchphrase at this, the potential launch of new life. On the other hand, Dr. M, his partner in the practice, is known to say cheerfully at the moment of detonation, "Swim, boys, swim."

I KEEP DRINKING champagne through the last week of December. The fact is I'm not ready to be pregnant and am banking on there being a few months of failed treatment for my mind to catch up with what my body is doing. As the year winds down and I scarcely look at the calendar, I joke to myself that if the IUI works, perhaps I'll have an abortion. My dad and Marion come over for Christmas and we—L, the baby and I—spend a lovely day with them just north of New York, at the house of Marion's daughter and her American family. A few days later, on my dad's seventieth birthday, they all come into town and L throws him a bowling party, with printed T-shirts and a group photo that she solicits the waiter to take and that I know my dad, in his Englishness, finds simultaneously wonderful and completely alarming.

The baby sleeps throughout, parked in his stroller a way back from the bowling lane, not even surfacing at the shriek from L as I lean in to kiss him with a mouth covered in wing sauce.

I have been emphatic to my dad that I am trying for this baby alone, but I know he thinks that eventually L and I will end up in a conventional arrangement—that this is a drawn-out interim stage that has somehow survived the birth of her own baby. He is too diplomatic to say this, but it is practically a generational impossibility for him to think otherwise. The person to go to for the alternative view is my mother's younger sister, Fay, a favorite among her siblings and the only person in her family I'm still in regular touch with. My aunt is well up to speed on news of L and the baby and, a few days after Christmas, I call her in Johannesburg to fill her in on my treatment.

"I think it's very enterprising," she says airily. My aunt has a couple of dicey ex-husbands in her past, as do most of my aunts. "If I could have had my children without having any of *them*," she says, "that would have been my preference." Which is, of course, what I knew she would say and is precisely why I rang in the first place.

These are the last days of frivolity. Two weeks into January, I get my period and, just like that, I sober up. I stop dissembling about needing more time to adjust. I switch to Coke at the bar. Overnight, the sense of what it is to throw money at something with no definite endpoint becomes sickeningly real and I can't believe I was so cavalier in the first place.

"OK," says L, who is calm and sensible in the face of my panic. "So you'll go another month and then you'll see."

"Early days," says Dr. B. We are in his office, where he is reviewing the results from the blood test. "Your hormone levels look good, everything looks good."

He exudes just the right ratio of confidence to uncertainty, but I still don't trust large parts of this process. Like all for-profit industries, the fertility industry is set up to serve multiple interests, and at the back of my mind I have the uneasy feeling that when there is room for interpretation of the data, fertility doctors are incentivized to err on the side of positivity. (In America, that is. In England, it is the opposite: cost rationalization means that if you want a third, free cycle of IVF on the NHS, you have to lobby like hell to prove that you're not a lost cause. I'm not sure which is worse in this instance, false hope or fatalism.) A doctor's optimism needn't even be cynical—it's human nature to want effort to be met with reward—but it makes it hard for me to get a sense of what we are actually talking about. When Dr. B says my levels are "good," does he mean good-good? Or does he mean good in the context of an overall bad business?

"The unknown variable is egg quality, right?" I say.

"Yes. Without IVF, there's no way for us to determine the quality of the eggs." We sit in silence for a moment and my face must fall because Dr. B gets up and goes to the Keurig machine in the corner of the room. "Coffee?"

"I thought I wasn't supposed to drink coffee." He returns with two cups.

"If you were drinking eight cups a day I might suggest you cut back. But otherwise it's just . . ."

"Needless masochism?"

"Exactly."

I have to smile. Ordinarily, I'm a big fan of needless masochism. Show me an opportunity to deny myself comfort and I will show you a happy woman. But after my meeting with the guru in London, I made myself promise I'd resist superstition. I wouldn't go nuts and buy raspberry tea, or start eating pineapple at certain points in the month, or sit in the Fertility Chair at work—a chair in the London office in which the last three women who'd sat had got pregnant. I would cut back on alcohol, but unless the doctor told me to, I wouldn't give up coffee or make any other adjustments, and I'm delighted when Dr. B approves. From then on, every time I go into the clinic, I carry a large cup of Starbucks, to ward off the evil eye of fertility mania.

In the weeks that follow, the rhythm of the clinic syncs with my own. The clientele grows familiar. There is the woman who comes in with her sister. There is the one who never looks up from her Black-Berry and complains at the desk about the clinic's late running. At eight a.m., half of us still have wet hair from the shower and several sit with their eyes shut until the nurse comes to fetch them. I had wondered in advance if there'd be hostility among us, because statistically if one woman gets pregnant it would seem to lessen the chances for the rest of us. But this isn't the case at all. With each passing week, we register one another's ongoing presence with smiles of quiet solidarity.

The worst thing about treatment at this stage is the time commitment. Timing is everything in fertility and if the timing is off—if your eggs aren't ready to drop on the day you go in for the insemination—you are sent home and told to return the next day. Even when the timing is right, there is a lot of hanging around. It is like having a second job, one with irregular shift patterns and a lot of strip searches. Here I am, at nine-thirty a.m. on yet another cold Thursday morning, longing to be at my desk drinking coffee but instead lying half naked in stirrups while four people peer up my fanjo.

"Imagine if, every week for a month, you went into an office so someone could stick something up your arse?" said a friend of mine to her husband recently when he implied that what she was going through for IVF wasn't that big of a deal. She said he looked a little shocked; the penny had finally dropped.

My actual job, meanwhile, gets crammed into the far corners of the day. It's an advantage of being almost forty and doing this that I can tread water for a while without fear of slipping. I can't imagine having had fertility treatment—or a baby, for that matter—during the years when I was still anxious about work. The only thing I hope is that no one cross-references the column I write with topics on the *Today* show, which in January through February become eerily aligned. Diets, fig-ure skaters, sleep studies, winter Olympic backgrounders; for six weeks Matt Lauer's producers do half of my work for me. (I never get a sin-gle idea from *TMZ;* thanks for nothing, guys.) The only items I don't take up are the ones about babies. When they come on-screen, which they do at regular intervals—cute babies, miracle babies, sick babies, talented babies—all the women in the waiting room laugh or make cooing sounds to puncture the awkwardness of ten strangers whose thoughts suddenly align. Then we spin off into our own thoughts again.

One Saturday midway through my second cycle, I go in for blood work, and because we're en route to Costco in her car, L comes in with me. If this story were Greek myth, going to Costco would stand in for our archetypal journey; some part of us is, has been and ever will be on the road to Costco. It's where we have our best conversations, looking not at each other but out of the window, absolved of the need to make eye contact. That morning, however, I'm anxious. When L brings the baby into the waiting room, it feels undiplomatic. (There are, I know, fertility clinics with signs on the walls asking visitors not to bring in their kids, which strikes me as even more embarrassing for the patients than the presence of an actual child, like having a sign up at a funeral home saying DON'T MENTION THE DEAD.) As it turns out, the other women couldn't be nicer, cooing and spoiling him, and then Dr. B comes out to shake L's hand and greet her warmly.

"That was weird," I say afterward, as we head out of town in the car.

"Yeah," she says.

It was quite touching, too, the efforts made by the doctor to chivy us together, and afterward, I feel bad for him. Then I feel bad for us. The failure, it seems to me, is less in the nature of our relationship than in our ability to give an adequate account of it, and as we wander around Costco, L pushing the cart, me hauling stuff into it, I wonder again how we look from the outside. Within a few weeks, Dr. B has stopped referring to "you both" in my posttreatment debriefs and started addressing his remarks uniquely to me.

"By the way," I say to him. It is a Friday morning, the final ultrasound before my second insemination.

"Hmmm?" he says, eyes on the screen.

"You never told me what the three Gs were."

His eyes zip across to meet mine and for a moment he looks at me, as if trying to figure out whether he can trust me. "Go on," I say.

"It's kind of a joke."

"What?"

"I'm not being entirely serious, so don't—."

"WHAT?"

He grins. "Guns, gold and a getaway plan."

. . .

A FEW DAYS LATER, I'm in the waiting room looking at the Christmas cards still tacked to the wall and texting Oliver a link to a piece about "sweat shaming." (It's for a fantasy Web site we operate called ThankYouForYourContribution.com, an anthology of the world's worst opinion pieces, and the fact that it exists only in our minds doesn't stop us from lovingly curating it.)

"Good luck today!" says Oliver. "If that is the appropriate statement of support. You may think luck has nothing to do with it."

"Thanks."

When I go into the treatment room, Olga, the nurse, is at the desk leafing through a large book. I like Olga. She has been working in IVF since the 1980s, at the very dawn of the technology, and is due to retire any day. A few weeks earlier, I'd been waiting to go into the ultrasound room and heard a woman crying on the other side of the door. "Ach, it can be hard," said Olga, with an air of deep tragedy I found somehow consoling. The expression on her face, which is etched with compassion, implied what does any of this matter, we'll all one day be dust.

The book Olga is reading is a photographic account of life inside the womb, featuring vivid color images of babies in utero and which, as I undress, she holds up to show me. I murmur appreciatively but inside I recoil. Those pictures of pink fetuses, curled over themselves like shrimp, have been so co-opted by the antiabortion lobby that you can't look at them now without visualizing some spit-flecked nutter waving a placard outside a clinic in Wichita. In any case, I don't want to think about the "miracle" of conception; the whole enterprise is improbable enough without adding a supernatural dimension to it. Olga shuts the book and we chat for a few moments before Dr. B comes in, followed by a nurse, who, once again, holds up the vial of sperm for my inspection. This checking protocol has been in place for two decades, ever since a lawsuit was brought against the clinic by a white couple who unexpectedly gave birth to a black child. "So you're waiting nine months to see if you'll have a baby of the wrong race," I say to Oliver later that day.

"Now, then, Brockesy," says Oliver. "I think we both know there's no such thing as the wrong race."

The procedure feels like nothing at all; a tiny bit of cramping and then, "Can you see them?" says Dr. B, indicating the screen. Sperm are, apparently, surging across my system like deer on the Serengeti.

"Oh, wow!" I say. (I can't see them.)

"All you have to remember is not to get your period!" He sweeps out of the room, taking the nurses with him.

You are supposed to keep still for ten minutes after the insemination and I lie in the semidarkness, looking up at the dusty collection of fertility dolls arranged on a shelf above the desk. One has a bow and arrow. One is dressed in some kind of folk costume. All look as if they have the potential to come alive at night. I think about the Christmas cards in the waiting room, which feature family photos from grateful former patients. That's nice, I think. All those success stories. Although there is something a little proprietorial about the montage, a little preening. From the clinic's point of view, I don't like the egotism of that wall—look at what we made!—and I don't like being lumped in with a bunch of people on the basis of fertility. This isn't a church, I think grumpily, it's a business; they should be grateful to me.

I don't know how long I'm lying there, but when Sophia, one of the nurses, comes back in she looks surprised to see me. "Hey," she says, tapping me lightly on the knee. "You can put your booty away now, honey."

I get up, redress, put on my snow boots which are standing in a puddle under a chair in the corner and leave the ultrasound room. On the way out, I glance at the wall of Christmas cards again and notice something I had failed to see earlier, even though it is the most prominent thing about the display: the sheer number of photos with more than one baby in them.

SEVEN

Drugs

IT IS THAT EVENING, a few hours after the insemination, that I feel
it starting to happen. At first, it is an impulse to wander up Atlantic
Avenue to the health-food store, just to see if they have it. Then, browsing the store's overlit aisles and failing to find anything, it is the urge to
run into Manhattan to the store on Fourteenth Street, no big deal, I'll be
back by nine p.m., it is pitch-black and raining but I have no other plans.
Then I find it (a sign!), pay twelve dollars—one buck per raspberry tea
bag, or "nature's aid to conception," as the packet informs me—and go
home to drink what tastes like a cup of hot flowers. By the end of the
week, I am going to the corner deli and buying precut pineapple that is
more expensive than flying to Puerto Rico and picking it myself.

This is how it begins. What harm can it do? Why *wouldn't* I try
everything? I mean, of course it won't work, but what if it does? I mean,
it won't, but what if it does? It won't. But what if it does? If athletes win

races based on a matter of milliseconds, mightn't raspberry tea close an even more infinitesimal gap? I have been trying to get pregnant for precisely six weeks but already I can glimpse the outline of the monster coming over the hill. Each failed attempt will get harder to shrug off. Expenses will mount. My life will go on being indefinitely on hold. Given this forecast, most of us would rather feel the shame of doing something illogical than the powerlessness of doing nothing at all.

"I bought the raspberry tea," I say to L on the phone later that night and wonder how she will take it. L believes in drugs not vitamins, but she has an unlikely artisanal streak. Long before classes at Fleishers, the butcher in Park Slope, became a staple gift item at Christmas, she wanted to learn how to butcher her own meat. She might look like a corporate American, but she'll buy cheesecloth to make her own yogurt. She almost certainly knows more about granola than you do. When we first met, one of my favorite things was to take her to a dinner party and watch her baffle the hipsters. "I'm proud of my country," she once said, startling the public radio producer to her left who'd just been banging on about how awful America is. He commenced sniggering, until L invited him to consider the possibility that if his family, like hers, had emerged from the concentration camps after the Second World War he mightn't take America for granted, either.

"You're an idiot," she says about the tea bags.

I retreat to my bed and my own form of patriotism: watching British sitcoms from the 1980s on YouTube, then calling up the opening credits to *Question Time*. (*Question Time*: a dowdy British panel show in which government ministers interact with awkward members of the public in a way that somehow sums up the essence of home. When I first came to the United States, one of the things I noticed was the ability of the average American to be stopped on the street, asked about practically anything and effortlessly summon a credible sound bite. There is something endearing about the average Briton's complete lack of competence when a microphone is shoved in his face.)

The fact is that within a week of the second insemination, I have caved in entirely to crank remedies and the crank rationalizations that go with them. I'm sure I feel little peckings in my abdomen and lie down for hours on my bed, willing the cells to divide. I avoid bending, shaking or making any sharp movements lest I kill the incipient baby. Online, I get tearful over cynical marketing campaigns.

"Is it terrible that I liked the Lily Allen / John Lewis Christmas song?" I ask my friend Leila by e-mail. It's a soppy ballad by a midlist pop star that ran over a Christmas commercial for a London department store—the equivalent of being moved by a billboard for Macy's.

"Fuckinlilyallenjohnlewis . . . you've gone proper expat."

A week later, Leila is stretched out in my living room, visiting from London for a few days while she hosts a panel at a human rights forum in the city. L and the baby have come down from Manhattan to have lunch with us and while L does things in the kitchen, Leila plays with the baby on the sofa. I watch them from across the room. It looks so simple, a woman playing with a baby. Not just a woman, but my friend, and not just any friend, but one of my oldest and best friends, interacting with L's baby with the kind of license and ease with which I would expect her to interact with my own.

There is a short story by Harold Brodkey called "The State of Grace," the last lines of which I think about that afternoon and return to a lot in subsequent days. In the story, Brodkey looks back on himself as a thirteen-year-old, babysitting a much younger child and shying away from the child's tacit request for affection. The last line, uttered in despair at the inadequacies of a life underlived, is "Love him, you damn fool, love him." I look at Leila, giggling with the baby on the sofa, and consider whether, in spite of the endless bickering between L and me, the constant anxiety over whether what we're doing is right, this is the last line. Is this only ever the last line? And if so, does it make what we're doing terrifically complicated, or incredibly simple? Love him, you damn fool, love him.

The fact is, I do love him, a little more each day. I can't say this too often to L; she gets tearful. I will discover this for myself one day—the profound effect of someone who doesn't "have" to love one's baby nonetheless going ahead and doing so. For now, however, it is simply astonishing. I have always had a lazy, negative reaction to adoption; too much hassle; too much heartbreak. Too much pressure to compensate for that primal rejection of the birth parents. I want to be pregnant for the experience of it and I want the child to be biologically mine for reasons of ego and as a link to my mother. But when I look at L's baby, with whom I have neither a genetic link nor any formal responsibility for, my heart judders to a degree I would never have thought possible. I look at Leila, who was adopted from an orphanage in India and raised in Britain by white people and is such a testament to the limitations of the genetic argument that my dad, who has known her as long as I have, once said, "I wish Leila was my daughter." ("All right, steady on," I said.)

Naïvely, perhaps, the risks inherent in my situation—of loving a baby I have no legal rights to—have never struck me as real, partly, I suspect, because I'm so distracted by the task of getting pregnant and partly because I've never considered him mine. It is hard to imagine a scenario in which L, who denies her son nothing, would deny him my love when I pose no threat to her parental rights. If our relationship has, at some level, been constructed to serve our needs as two single parents, then the biggest threat to us now isn't some fight over the baby, but what happens if I fail to get pregnant.

"YOU CAN'T CAUSE a miscarriage from jogging," says Leila. It's the following morning. She is lying on an airbed in my living room, surrounded by wardrobe options.

"I don't need to dress up, do I?" I'd said when she invited me to come with her to the human rights forum—oh, OK, it was the U.N.—that afternoon.

"No. But don't wear your fleece."

"I'm not going to wear my fleece. If I stick up my hand, will you take my question about Syria?"

"Assuming it's not 'Where is Syria?'"

Leila has almost no tolerance for the nonsense around fertility and, in spite of the icy temperatures, suggests we do something to burn off her nerves and give me a feeling of agency, which is to take ourselves out for a run. A few years earlier, I'd spent hundreds of dollars on sneakers and thermal base layers, even doing a race organized by the New York Road Runners club and feeling sufficiently invested to be vain about my time. For my last birthday, Leila got me a personalized message from the guy who makes the Couch to 5K app, which I'd picked up at the airport and made me squeal while boarding a flight to Miami. Since then, I've lapsed, but Leila hasn't. I look out of the window; there is still snow on the ground.

"Um," I say. For a moment, the two halves of my new personality—the one that wants to give in to the madness and the rational side—clash. "OK."

We run east toward the river, our breath coming out in thin clouds, then carry on all the way to the Brooklyn Bridge. I start out mincing, clenching my uterus to prevent the zygote from joggling out of its seat, but after fifteen minutes I forget and just run. "See?" she says. "It isn't so bad."

It isn't so bad. I should feel good. I have overcome superstition and done something healthy. For some reason, however, it doesn't feel like a victory. On my own in the flat later, I consider my frazzled state and can't help feeling that just this once, I should have asserted my right to be weak, even at the expense of spooking my friend.

On the other hand, as the end of the month approaches, I am increasingly convinced that good news is on its way and, as a result, am extravagantly casual about my chances. On the phone to my dad I chatter about the curried goat I had for lunch at a restaurant in Midtown and tell him about L's baby's hilarious language gaffs. I go on about my nostalgia for Britain, which makes my dad laugh and tell me I've been out of the country for too long; the Tories, slashing NHS budgets and flogging off large parts of the capital to foreign billionaires, have turned the place into a mini-America.

"Any news?" he says tentatively at the end of the call.

"No!!" I say, with the manic cheer of a hippie about to go mad with an ax. I don't say, "At thirty-eight? With no drugs? On the second try? Are you insane?" but my tone implies it, expertly setting up an expectation of failure against which my forthcoming victory will be all the more stunning. A few days later, Leila goes home. A few days after that, I get my period. So much for fucking raspberry tea.

All my warm feelings about adoption, about L's baby potentially being "enough" and about love being all we need evaporate in a flash. The cold, sharp edge of competition rises to a shriek in my soul. At the very best, at this point, I may turn out to be statistically average. At the very worst, I may prove irredeemably defective. This has nothing to do with wanting a baby. This is about winning and losing. There is only one possible bright side to my failure this month and that is if I *had* been pregnant, I would have had to rearrange my entire mental landscape to accommodate the possibility that herbal remedies actually work. As it is, I return to the clinic, disappointed by the growing evidence that I'm not exceptional and carrying a cup of Starbucks the size of my head.

Dr. B makes himself coffee and returns to his seat. His expression is one of mild wryness, as if the human condition were one in which he and I take a mutual but largely dispassionate interest. He recommends Clomid, an oral drug designed to stimulate the ovaries and trick my body into releasing more than one egg the following month, before moving on to discuss the American government's manipulation of the international money markets.

My body doesn't respond to the Clomid, and a month later, I produce a single egg that fails to fertilize. Three failures. Three months. Five thousand dollars and counting.

There is a photo of me taken around that time that captures the state I am in. It is early February and it is snowing again, the kind of laborious New York snow that looks as if it were falling upward. A photographer from the *New York Times* has come to my apartment to do a portrait for a piece about family secrets, to which I have contributed some thoughts about my mother. We do a few setups, some in my office, some in the living room in front of the bookcase, where, I realize too late, a book called *Dateworthy: Get the Relationship You Want* is on prominent display behind my head. "If that ends up in the *Times* I'm going to fucking kill you," I say to L, who forced the book on me in the first place. But the photo they end up using is worse, in a way, a classic local newspaper shot of Miserable-Looking Woman Stares Into Camera While Holding Up Photo Of Dead Person. "It's not that bad," says L doubtfully when it comes out a few weeks later. But it is. I look utterly dejected.

"I don't get the sense that statistically anything out of the ordinary has happened yet," says Oliver. And while I can see this is true, for once the rationalizations don't work. It still feels like a personal failure.

I don't call Merope, or Kate, my best-friend-from-college, who have two children apiece and neither of whom, I think, can possibly understand. And I don't tell my dad, whose anxiety hurts me more than my own. Instead, I go online to the infertility forums, those groups and comment threads in which women struggling to get pregnant hang out. I have heard about these from friends and know no good can come of consulting them, but I don't care. Stoicism hasn't worked. Now I want to wallow.

As it turns out, I have no idea what I'm getting into. Page after page of women discussing their reproductive histories going back eight, nine, ten failed cycles, volumes of treatment I didn't even know it was possible or legal to have. Some have been TTC (trying to conceive) for twelve years, a struggle many of them itemize in an e-mail kicker, so that with every glib posting their entire traumatic backstory republishes. I scroll down in horror; contributors listing every drug they have taken and the dates they found out they weren't pregnant, or worse, when they conceived and lost the baby. The tone of the postings is one of fake cheer, with a sense of clubby exceptionalism that comes from using the jargon. Having fertility treatment is a little like taking out your first mortgage and getting a buzz from saying things like "marginal interest rate" or "discretionary ARM," only in this case it's "gonadotropin," and "follicle," and "endometrium," and "hypoestrogenic." I had done this myself and considered it harmless. Now, however, I can see how dangerously seductive this superficial expertise is, how it keeps hope alive and confers on each woman a tenuous sense of control. Infinitely sadder is the jolly shorthand—for the results of a pregnancy test, BFN (big fat negative) and BFP (big fat positive); DH for darling husband; all the way down to EWCM, for egg white cervical mucus—that users clearly think communicates cavalier good humor but (is this how I seem to others?) instead just looks flagrantly unhinged.

No one shows signs of wanting to give up or move on. No one has a prognosis so bad that someone somewhere in the group hasn't heard of another woman in the same situation who still managed to get pregnant. Rather than wishing one another luck, everyone wishes one another sprinkles of "baby dust," at which point I get off the site and make myself promise never to go back.

And so, to anyone reading this who is in the early stages of fertility treatment, I offer some advice: before you get in too deep, write down where your cutoff is, whether that be three rounds of IVF, a fifty-thousand-dollar spend, or a year of trying. Write it in big letters and stick it to your fridge door, along with a printout of your bank statement, a list of everything you love about your life and possibly a copy of your marriage certificate. Write a list of all the acronyms you never want to find yourself using, and the number of jaunty exclamation points beyond which someone needs to reach in and pull you out.

Better yet, prearrange an intervention from friends and family. Because once you're in it, all reason will fly out the door. You will buy the raspberry tea. You will eat the pineapple. You will sit in the Fertility Chair at work (and that April, on a trip back to London, I do). You will fall down the rabbit hole into the infertility forums and anyone who questions you will be given the kind of short shrift you give a friend who tries to cut you off after your third martini. Meanwhile, the bar will keep serving you until you throw up.

Well beyond that point, in fact; until you are taken away in an ambulance, put on a drip and required to sell all your assets to settle the bar tab.

SO HERE WE ARE, month four. Time for the heavy artillery. Repronex, Fertinex, Follistim: they sound like gynecological problems that would have interested Freud. In fact, they are brand names belonging to the next stage of fertility drugs. If Clomid, a synthetic drug, works by triggering an overproduction of the body's own hormones, then these drugs, known collectively as gonadotropins, are identical to the hormones produced in the brain and act directly on the ovaries to increase egg supply. They have a much higher success rate, with higher risks, but if this is explained to me, I don't hear it. One morning in March, I stand in Dr. B's office while a nurse unpacks a silver bag onto the table, containing swabs, syringes, needles and a handful of glass bottles, on the side of which is a name that doesn't immediately betray its usage. Bravelle: it could be a fancy private school or a yoga retreat in upstate New York.

There are clinics that make patients go in for a five-hour seminar on how to give themselves injections, but not this one. In five minutes flat, the nurse shows me how to load the syringe from the silver-capped bottle, deposit the liquid into the green one, shake to dissolve and load it back into the syringe. "Then change the needle and inject it here," she says, indicating a triangle below my belly button. I nod, grateful for her matter-of-factness, and figure I can look it all up on the Internet afterward. Then I cross the street to the pharmacy and hand over my pre-scription.

"Insurance?" says the pharmacist.

"Doesn't cover these drugs." (You would never in these circumstances say "I don't have insurance." You might, at a pinch, say "Self-pay," which implies resources so vast insurance isn't an issue. I have heard people do this: talk about expensive procedures they've had and then casually let drop that their doctor "doesn't take insurance." This means they're so wealthy, they don't need health insurance because what's a trifling ninety thousand dollars between a woman and her back surgeon?)

The pharmacist looks at me expectantly. I am still so stupid in the ways of the American system, I have no idea what her problem is.

"That'll be eighteen hundred dollars," she says in a voice designed not to carry.

"You're fucking joking." This comes out like a Tourette's outburst, guttural and spontaneous. The pharmacist blinks behind large specta-cles. "Here's a voucher that will get you two hundred dollars off," she says and we stand for a moment in silence, looking at each other over the two-dollar items on display at the cash register. Then I hand over my credit card.

One of the things the nurse has told me is that for psychological reasons, it can be easier to ask someone else to do the injection. "Come round," says L on the phone that afternoon, "I'll do it."

"You will not." I once let her cut my hair after she'd watched a video on YouTube and was convinced she knew how to do layers and although, to be fair, it was as good as some $150 haircuts I've had, there was some-thing off about the symmetry that I don't fancy seeing translated into puncture wounds in my belly. If any amateur is going to stab me with a needle, it'll be me, and that evening, after watching an instructional video put out by the drug company, I lay the paraphernalia out on my desk and immediately run up against the first problem.

Have you ever actually looked at your abdomen? Where does it start and your torso stop? Or your "side"? How big are the ovaries and where exactly are they? What if I miss the spot and, as with the hero in *James and the Giant Peach,* throw magic at the wrong thing? Will I blow up my appendix? Or poison my liver? It's not that I'm squeamish. I could never be a doctor or skin a rabbit, but I don't run screaming from the sight of blood. And I'm not frightened of the pain. It's more the prospect of messing it up—of doing the fertility-drug equivalent of Woody Allen sneezing away the cocaine in *Annie Hall.* This stuff is so expensive that if I cock up a single injection, overdilute it or drop it and shatter the vial, I will have to buy a whole new course of treatment.

Eventually, after injecting liquid in and out of the syringe multiple times, rewatching the video and satisfying myself that the air bubble is too small to kill me, I settle on a target and stand holding the needle an inch from my belly. Do it. Do it. Do it. Can't do it. Do it. Can't do it. DO IT. Can't do it. For god's sake do it.

I carefully lay down the syringe, walk to the kitchen, pull out a packet of frozen peas from the freezer, slam it against my flank and hold it there until the area goes numb. Then I go back to my office and ram the needle in up to the hilt. It doesn't hurt at all. I am euphoric.

From then on, I look forward to the injection all day: wiping the lunch crumbs from my desk and disinfecting the surface; laying out the gear; twisting on the big needle, mixing in the liquid, twisting on the little needle, then flicking the syringe and jabbing it in. Nothing about drug use has ever appealed to me, except what I can now see is the power of the ritual. There is something mesmerizing about going through the same drill every day. Sometimes I am heavy-handed with the needle and a dark bead of blood forms on the surface of the skin. Sometimes I get in and out cleanly. Then I deposit the needle in the toxic-waste receptacle given to me by the clinic and swab the area clean, feeling as if I've just performed six hours of brain surgery.

It never crosses my mind to think about what is in the drugs, although I've since read that it's a derivative of urine, specifically, the urine of postmenopausal women, which contains high levels of the hormones that stimulate egg production. This makes sense, I guess, that the aging female body responds to the dearth of eggs by producing larger and larger amounts of the hormone responsible for producing them. Anyway, at the time I couldn't be less interested. As with all drugs, I assume it is awful and toxic and that, save for the reason I am taking it, I would be better off not taking it. What can I do? It could be George's Magic Medicine for all I cared as long as it does its job.

"You're responding very well to the drugs," says Dr. B a couple of weeks later. This sounds like good news, but he looks uneasy. We are in his office after the ultrasound, which has revealed I am on course to produce more eggs in a month than the average woman produces in an entire year. I envisage them stacked up like bombs in a World War II airplane, my poor, laboring ovaries cranking out one after another after another. If a woman is born with a finite number of eggs, and if, like rings on an oak, every egg dropped represents a month of her life, then I have a gynecological age of about ninety-seven at this point.

"Frankenstein," I say jokingly and Dr. B looks irritated in the same way a friend of mine did when I asked him how many people he'd had to bribe to get his property business in the Balkans off the ground.

"Not Frankenstein," he says and I can see him turning the word over in his mind. "We'll cut the dosage. But . . ."

I don't want to hear it. I'm not interested in the risks. I don't even know what they are, beyond some vague threat of "overstimulating" the ovaries, which was, I thought, the whole point of the exercise. After the failures of the past few months, all I can hear is that I have responded well; more than well, exceptionally! If you had told me, a year earlier, that a large chunk of my self-esteem would rest on how many eggs my ovaries could be artificially stimulated into producing in a given month, I would have thought you were mad. Now here I am, strutting around feeling great about myself on account of my MASSIVE EGG STASH. Suddenly, I understand why men go in for penis enlargements.

"How's your jizzing?" says my friend Janice later that week. "I've been worrying about it." We are at the bar at Blue Ribbon Sushi on Columbus Circle, eating bone marrow rice. ("Jizz," as well as being a slang term for sperm, serves as shorthand for the kind of high-turnover journalism we both work in and to which we occasionally refer as "jism." Anyway, she meant the other jizzing.) I wince.

"It's fine," I say. "No big deal."

"Is it painful, when they do it?"

"Nope. They just wazz it up your fanjo and off you go."

I tell her, boastfully, that I have "overresponded" to the drugs and am carrying a ton of eggs around in my midsection, and after laughing, Janice, who is British, shakes her head and says, "This country is insane."

I hadn't thought to look at it that way. It's true that if I was at home, where public health policy recommends only "small doses of fertility drugs" for IUI patients, I would almost certainly not be in the position I'm in. But while I laugh with my friend at the reckless Americans, I'm secretly, almost hysterically, grateful. It might be alarming to have produced a high-bordering-on-insane number of eggs this month, but it is surely preferable to the miserly alternative. If I want a result, these are the breaks. I want a result. I will take my chances.

The following Saturday, I lug my giant egg hoard back to the clinic for the insemination. It is their busiest time of the week and the place is teeming. L and I are, once again, en route to Costco and while she waits for me outside in the car, I sit in the waiting room anxiously watching the clock. Because of the rush, appointments are running way behind schedule, and when I finally get into the treatment room, the atmosphere is so harried and unpleasant that Dr. B rushes in and starts conducting the ultrasound, without raising a single concern about the secret world order.

"I have to ask you," he says, frowning at the screen. "How do you feel about high-order multiples?" This is the first time I have heard the term.

"What do you mean?"

"Three or more."

I burst out laughing. "Three or more babies?! I don't feel good about that."

"I'm serious."

"So am I. I don't feel good about that."

It may strike you as absurd that I haven't considered this sooner. But I haven't. All I have done for a straight fortnight is preen about my egg supply and speculate on how it elevates my chances of getting pregnant this month. In spite of the Christmas card wall, in spite of a million tabloid stories about fertility treatment gone awry, it simply hasn't occurred to me that the chances of getting too pregnant are part of the deal. This is particularly true when you have IUI. In an IVF cycle, doctors stimulate the ovaries to produce a large number of eggs, then remove them and, after fertilizing them outside of the body, decide how many embryos to transfer back into the woman. In the UK, by law, a maximum of two embryos can be transferred to a women under forty and three to a woman over forty; in the United States, by guideline, up to three embryos for the under forties, and five for the over forties.

With IUI, there is no control over how many eggs fertilize. Once you've taken the drugs, all bets are off. This is how Jon and Kate Gosselin got into their situation. Their sextuplets weren't a result of wanton use of IVF, but of standard IUI, of triggering ovulation in a woman who has produced large numbers of eggs and decides to go ahead with the insemination anyway. Some doctors will cancel a cycle if more than four or five eggs mature in time for ovulation. Others will press ahead, because it's impossible to tell how many of those eggs are viable. The implications of producing "too many" eggs, and how many are too many, are notoriously difficult to judge.

"It's up to you," says the doctor and looks at me. The nurses look at me. Everybody looks at me and waits. For the first time, I feel a twinge of fury. Can they really be raising this for the first time now, at the eleventh hour? For god's sake I've already taken my pants off. And of course I can't bring myself to do it—to throw away the cycle, waste more than two thousand dollars and start all over again the following month, not to mention face the embarrassment of telling everyone in the room to stand down.

"Go ahead," I say grimly.

"OK." He flicks a look at a nurse, who turns to the tray and picks up the catheter. "With this many eggs, you're going to feel a lot of cramps tomorrow."

By the time I come out, L has a parking ticket and we fight all the way to Costco. For the next five days I am in a terrible mood. On Thursday night, I dream of blood gushing out of me, and on Friday morning, when I get up to go to the loo, that is exactly what happens. Not just blood, but lumps. I am still bleeding on Sunday, when L and I drive out to Queens on an errand. While she talks to the guy about changing the oil in the car, I stand on the garage forecourt and feel the sky spin above me. I have let myself down. I have let Dr. B down, not just by failing to get pregnant but by failing to keep up my side of the bargain to be rational and not crumble and care. I thought I had this thing down but instead, here I am, malfunctioning at every possible level.

Dr. B is gloomy when I go in to report this on Monday. A pregnancy could potentially survive this kind of blood loss, he says, but it is unlikely, and after giving me a bunch of free samples of a drug designed to strengthen the lining of the womb, he suggests that if I fail to conceive with this many eggs, we can assume the egg quality is compromised. The analogy he makes, unkindly as it feels at the time, is with a "bum coin": after throwing it a bunch of times and getting the same result, the probability of a new outcome lessons with each throw until it whittles down to zero.

Then he says a word to strike fear into my heart: "escalation."

"I would try one, or at most two, more cycles of IUI," says Dr. B.

"Two," I blurt, finally getting the hang of second-guessing my doctors. It has been only four months. If I was under NHS care, I would potentially have to go through ten—ten!—failed cycles of IUI before being diagnosed with "unexplained infertility" and qualifying for the next stage. I'm not ready to start paying ten thousand dollars a throw for IVF, nor to admit that I have a real problem. Dr. B gives me a small shrug; OK, on your head be it.

The following day, I have a dental appointment and shuffle miserably to the clinic in Park Slope. I love my dentist. It's the kind of place I used to go as a child, with faded twenty-five-year-old prints of art exhibitions on the wall and an aggressively unglamorous waiting room. As the dentist loads up the anesthetic for the filling, I mumble something about being pregnant.

"What was that?" she says.

"There's a small possibility I might be pregnant but probably not." I must go bright red because she stares at me. "OK, well, if there's even a small chance you're pregnant, I wouldn't be happy injecting you." She puts down the needle, cancels the work and doesn't charge for the visit. "It can be hard," she says kindly as I leave the room. On the way out, I go to the loo, stare at my reflection in the chrome surface of the hand-towel dispenser and burst into tears. And there you have it; the worst has happened. I've become the woman crying in a public toilet about her ovaries. I go home, type "heavy blood loss + still pregnant" into the infertility forum and give myself up to an afternoon of self-loathing.

AT NO POINT, either then or in the days that follow, do I consider throwing in the towel. I have invested too much time and energy to walk away with nothing. L is calm and encouraging and thinks the doctor is too keen to move on, although I suspect there is something noble in his calculation that IVF might save me time and money at this point. Anyway, L's steadiness is soothing, and for a second I wonder if this is what it is like to let someone else carry half of the load.

There is a single good thing to come out of the month. After you've taken fertility drugs, persisting with the delusion that raspberry tea makes a difference is like dropping an H-bomb, then sending in a man with a cutlass, and just like that, I let the woo-woo stuff go. I think about advice from the coast guard about what to do if you get caught in a rip tide—overcome the instinct to struggle and give yourself up to the current, so that in due course, with any luck, you will wash up bedraggled but alive on some distant shore. Finally, I understand that no amount of industry on my part will change how this thing turns out. When it comes to functions of the body, there is only blood and luck.

The next day, I am due to fly to Vancouver for work. "I think you should cancel," says L. I am still bleeding heavily and my insurance is iffy, claiming it won't cover complications arising from fertility treatment.

"Yeah, but it's Canada," I say. "They look after you there." At five a.m., I go to the airport carrying enough wadding to man a field hospital in Crimea. The bleeding continues steadily over the Midwest and during our descent into Vancouver's metropolitan area, although I feel better once I get to the hotel and install myself in Starbucks for an afternoon's work. My eggs might be hurling themselves like lemmings from the cliff. I might be about to throw my life savings down on a bet. But I can still cross a continent and efficiently meet a deadline on the other side. And at least I am getting away from that fucking clinic for a week. Even if it is my choice to be there.

EIGHT

Waiting

THERE IS SOMETHING my mother used to say about what would happen to her if something happened to me. This was, I understood, the only context in which it was OK to give up or fall apart, to be anything less than invincible. "If something happened to you," she would say blithely, "I would become an alcoholic." She took a little license with the grammar in that statement, given the amount she drank toward the end of her life. Nonetheless, I understood what she was saying. My mother, graduate of a terrible childhood, a woman who remade herself from scratch in her twenties and whose entire sense of self rested on being the person who doesn't collapse in the face of calamity, was boasting of her annihilation as a marker of how much she loved me. There was, she meant to imply, nothing bigger in the universe than a mother's love for her child and no devastation greater than the event of her losing it. Which was all well and good. But what of this: the devastation of losing a child one never had? What of losing the idea of oneself as a mother? What is the appropriate response then?

Here is the paradox and perhaps the cruelest thing about fertility treatment: that the harder I engage in trying to have a child, the more I want one, and the harder it becomes to convince myself of something I once took for granted—that I'll be absolutely fine if I don't. The term "baby hunger," which has always offended me as infantilizing, in a similar category of insult to that of saying women can't be presidents or prime ministers because they are erratic for five days of the month, is now an accurate description of how I feel. I am manic, ravenous, clawing at the door of motherhood begging to be let in, terrified of what will happen if I'm not.

I have always been able, through a little mental effort, to sell myself on the idea that whatever happens is the very thing I wanted to happen in the first place—I'm not married; I don't care, I like my own space; I don't have a banker-size salary; fine, an interesting job is more important than money—but there is nothing I can do with not being able to have children, no story I can tell that will make it OK. Of all the competing types of shame in my system, this is by far the worst, having to admit to myself I have been wrong all these years. I think back to how I scoffed at the older woman in my office, the one who broke rank to lecture me about not waiting too late to have children. I think of all my protestations of what it is to have a meaningful life—that work is the thing, that education is the thing, that travel and culture and friends are the thing, that connection to another adult human being is the thing, all of which, it turns out, and as I have known all along, are, if not secondary, then at the very least weaker delivery systems for the main business of life, if one believes that business to be love. It's wrong and reductive to value a woman on whether she has children, but in terms of the way I value my own life, the idea of their absence, now that I'm forced to confront it, feels like an extinction-level event.

I am in Vancouver to cover the annual TED conference and, after returning from Starbucks, stand in the chintzy hotel room and taunt myself with the prospect of this being my life for the rest of my life: a string of loosely connected anecdotes leading nowhere and building to nothing. I'll carry on meeting deadlines in foreign cities, then head out to find junk food. I'll lie in bed until noon on Sunday mornings, a vast and terrible array of choices before me, none requiring my attention more urgently than the next. I will grow even more petulant about not getting my way, because my own way will be all I have to consider. My life will take on a different shape to that of my friends with children, stripped of all those petty concerns that I know, from my own mother's death, when nothing hurt more than finding scraps of old notes from her or chipped buttons she had sewn into my clothes, add up to a greater sum than their parts. I will hold myself to account in ways that can only add to my shame, the calculation being, particularly for women, that if you don't have the baby you wanted, you'd jolly well better have something else to show for it, and nothing short of a Nobel Prize or the best, most passionate relationship will do.

That last one terrifies me. I have never regarded being in a couple as an end in itself, either for form's sake or because I hate being alone. Even in the early days with L, when I was as in love with her as I've been with anyone, it struck me that being with someone is basically a nightmare a lot of the time. I've always rather despised women who are never single and boast of how they haven't dated since they were sixteen because of all their wonderful long-term relationships. What's wrong with them? I thought. Why is their sense of self so vested in being with somebody else?

Now all of this flies out the window. Without a child, I'll have to get one of those relationships in which we grow old together and finish off each other's sentences and start looking as alike as dogs and their owners—certainly not the relationship I have with L, whose priority is her baby and who I am, by any metric, wrong for in about twenty-four different categories. No one, looking at us, would mistake us for the perfect couple, or even for a couple at all half the time. If my relationship is going to make up for not having children, then I'll have to get back into the dating pool, and of everything, I think, this is the most depressing consideration of all. Have a baby, and I will potentially never have to wash my hair again. Don't have a baby, and I will have to keep primping and preening and shaving my legs as I get older and my stock withers and dies.

One of the advantages of my job is that it proffers a million opportunities to lose oneself in someone else's concerns, and just as these thoughts are becoming unbearable, I leave the hotel to head out for the conference. Vancouver is a beautiful city full of wide, light-drenched streets and views across great sheets of water. At the convention center, which overlooks Vancouver harbor, I pick up my huge ID badge and the gift bag allocated to every attendee. (It contains a combination of small luxuries—coconut water and KIND bars—and things you can't get hold of in the normal run of things, like TED-branded bags and water bottles. I have a collection of ugly items from around the world in this vein, including an EU-branded beach towel from a summit in Thessaloniki, a woolly hat from the NATO gift shop in Kosovo and a pin from a donkey sanctuary in Kashmir, all trinkets that bring back happy memories and remind me to celebrate the day I stopped saying yes to everything.)

TED, as most people know, started out as a modest tech and design forum and exploded over the years into a franchise styled as the world's greatest minds tackling the world's hardest problems to a paying audience of the world's richest arseholes and I have to say, if one must endure the sudden exit from one's system of two dozen unfertilized eggs, there are worse places in which to do it. The toilets are clean. There are stunning views over the water. As I wander around the conference hall, Al Gore is never far from my peripheral vision. There are coffee stations and yoga stations and a confectionary stand that doesn't dispense candy but is committed to "storytelling through chocolate." On a communal white board, someone has written "ohmygod we are soooo lucky to be here," and someone else, "a drawing is simply a line going for a walk," all of which I write down with a view to making fun of later before retiring for an hour to the toilets.

The theme of the conference is, loosely, resilience, and while people might say they attend TED for the wacky serendipity of ideas, really what resilience means in this context is how to maximize one's performance at work. It's what links the scientist who, after studying the unique motor abilities of cockroaches, found a way to replicate their movements in robotic form with the guy who dragged a sled to the Antarctic and the woman who developed software to thwart cyberattacks. More broadly, it represents what feels to me like the American style of striving for success without concealing one's efforts. I remember years ago, Merope calling me on a Monday morning to say she felt guilty for not getting more done on the weekend, to which I said something pious like not everything has to have measurable results. I believed this at the time, and still do, but only because of some weaselly inner logic which argues that the *real* way to make something happen is to allow for the possibility that it won't. "The slack line catches the biggest fish," wrote Thomas McGuane in his memoir of fishing and writing, a principle I believe in with a kind of superstitious fervor: stop trying so hard—or rather, stop appearing to try so hard—and you will get what you want. Allow yourself to fail—or rather, allow it to appear that failure doesn't faze you—and only then will you prosper.

When I come out of the toilets it's almost five p.m. and getting dark. I'm not going to get pregnant. The thought strikes me with the force of a blow to the head. It's not for the best. There's no "teachable moment." It is simply the truth of my situation and for a moment, standing on the steps of the convention hall in the cool Canadian air, I feel high on the novelty of letting it go. I leave the center and cross the road to McDonald's, where I order a Quarter Pounder with cheese and sit at a table with a woman in a misshapen brown jacket, with whom I trade life-is-terrible vibes. I start to cheer up.

When I get outside again, a small crowd has gathered in front of the convention center to watch a light installation being switched on and in the crowd I spot a face that I recognize. Rosemary! It has been seven months since I saw her in Edinburgh, since when she has changed jobs and moved countries. We embrace, screaming.

"World's biggest name tag," I say, holding up my ID badge.

Rosemary makes a somber face and holds up her own. "By this lanyard shall ye know me."

I know Rosemary hasn't done anything yet about starting fertility treatment and I don't want to discourage her by sharing my news. I have been so committed to the idea of getting pregnant on the sly and presenting it as a brilliant fait accompli that I want to keep my failures to myself. I sense in my friend a similar reluctance to bring up the subject, and although I'm relieved, I'm sad, too. We have entered that no-man's-land in which small variables between women of late childbearing age feel like unbridgeable gulfs, and until we're on the other side of it, there is no point in trying to meet each other halfway. Instead, we talk about how sheepish we feel to be attending the conference without having invented a nanotechnology.

The truth is, I have spent the last four months pushing what I think of as the boundary between biology and technology, which in this company is laughable. Here, the anxiety about progress isn't should we, but could we. "How cool is this?" is justification enough. The following day, at the buffet—a presentation of deli meats that, mercifully, doesn't ask us to interrogate and reinvent the concept of lunch—I meet a woman who tells me she is a neuroscientist for a "stealth unit" at Google, working on "how to download human thought." There are others, too, all brilliant, all potentially world changing, but whose efforts strike me, in my febrile state, as so much window dressing on the primary unfathomability of how to be alive in one's body. Surely the only point of progress is to find new, more reliable ways in which to deliver the old certainties? This isn't a story about technology; it's a story about love.

I like the firefly expert. I like the guy who says, "I realized for the first time that light has substance and can be designed."

"Is it terrible that the thing I liked most was Billy Collins's poem about the dog?" says Rosemary. We are on a late afternoon break, vaguely stalking Larry Page around the auditorium perimeter.

"No. I liked it, too." Collins, the former U.S. poet laureate, had come onstage in sneakers and a red fleece and in a gruff, untheatrical voice recited a poem with no motivational value whatsoever about a dog anticipating its death.

I think about the brilliance of the mechanical cockroach; of how in order to replicate life, one must be able to break it down into its constituent parts, and of how the poets do this in arguably harder terms than the scientists. The big word at these conferences is "disruption," but it can be a narrow understanding of what form that might take. Satire, for example, is a disruptive force that, like the proverbial dog whistle, can't be heard by those who favor the exclamatory mode. Might not the poem about a dog be as powerful, in its way, as the blueprint for how to download a thought? Isn't that all a good poem is, anyway?

When my phone goes off, I leave Rosemary and walk through the heavy glass doors out onto the terrace.

"Is your head itching?" says L. I snap out of my reverie.

"You're joking."

"It's probably a false alarm."

"You are fucking joking."

My head instantly starts itching like crazy. "Fucking Melanie," I say. L, the baby and I had been to a friend's house the previous weekend and she'd sworn blind her kids' nit outbreak was under control.

"We've done the treatment just in case. You need to go to a pharmacy and buy the stuff."

Fifteen feet away, Al Gore stands looking out across the water, talking on his cell phone.

"How far do these things jump?"

IT'S NOT THAT I regret not having started out sooner. I'm not so lost as to believe that my younger self could have handled this; in fact, it seems to me the only thing worse than my present predicament would have been to be in my present predicament but with fewer resources. Neither do I wish I had frozen my eggs, a proposition that strikes me as ludicrous. The ideal time to freeze one's eggs, like the ideal time to start preparing for one's retirement, is in one's twenties, when it seems as if it will never be relevant. Nevertheless, I have two friends in their midthirties who are looking into the possibility of freezing their already quite elderly eggs, with a view to buying themselves another ten years to find a man. (Interestingly, both are confident their families will pay for it. Where parents once labored to cover their thirtysomething's wedding, now they're on the hook for their thirtysomething's egg-freezing operation. "They have to do it," said a friend the other day, "because they gave my sister a shit-ton for her problems, so they owe me. And anyway, otherwise they're not going to get grandkids.")

Besides, I like the focusing element of working to deadline. The shelf life of a woman's reproductive system is generally perceived to be a bad thing, but there is something to be said for being forced to prioritize. Meanwhile, men can drift on for years, messing up themselves and everyone else in the process. If I am unambivalent about wanting children, I am equally unambivalent about the value of the years I've spent not having them.

What I'm not prepared for is the complete lack of a plan as to how my life might look in their absence. Having kids in one's late thirties or early forties coincides almost exactly with the first sniff of midlife crisis, which is good if the baby thing works out. There is nothing like new life to defer one's encroaching decrepitude. If I don't have a baby, however, those years just got harder. I'll have more time on my hands, in which case, like any surplus resource, the value of that time will fall, and with it, somehow, the value of whatever comes out of it. If I do have a baby, on the other hand, I will create a background condition in which I am forced to be sharper and more resourceful than if I had to provide only for myself. I want a baby for all the reasons mentioned, but I also want a baby because I function best when there is some kind of resistance to overcome. Having a child is supposed to undermine one's ability to work, but that's not how I see it. In the tiny chamber of my brain dedicated to pure self-advancement, I think a baby will maximize my performance.

But I'm not having a baby. I have a job to do, followed by another. When I leave the conference in Vancouver a night early, missing Sting's keynote speech ("Ah, shame," says Rosemary), it is to fly down to San Francisco for a meeting at Facebook and at eleven p.m. I check into a roadside motel in Palo Alto. The balmy air feels outlandish after the deep cold of Vancouver. Perhaps Americans feel this way when they check into a bed-and-breakfast in the Lake District or a Travelodge off the A412—wholly invisible—and, as I tend to in these places, I fantasize about dropping out to live here for months, like a medieval mystic or a stylite up a pole: silent, sexless, anonymous, dreamless, stripped of all impurity and baggage. I don't need to be a mother. I don't need to be anything. I just need to get under these boiled white sheets and, with the sound of crickets bleeping in the warm air outside, sleep more deeply than I have done for weeks.

The next morning, I take a cab to the Facebook campus. I am interviewing Sheryl Sandberg for the paperback release of *Lean In,* in advance of which every woman with kids I know has urged me to find out how many nannies she has, what time she leaves the house in the morning and how many hours of the day she spends with her children relative to working—all inquiries that, it turns out, she not only is disinclined to answer but knocks back as fundamentally hostile to feminism. Men don't get asked these questions, so why should she? It's a rationale I've been hearing since I was twenty-two and made the mistake of asking one of Britain's foremost feminists about juggling "work and children," whereupon she looked at me over her half-moon spectacles in a way that ensured I never asked that question again.

At least, I never asked it directly. Instead, I insinuated it every which way. I have asked women about "guilt" and time management. I have asked actresses if they take their kids with them on set, and novelists if it's hard to shut the door. I have asked if motherhood has "changed" them, not a question that ever solicits an interesting answer, but one that, for most publications, is pretty much insisted on when a high-profile woman has children. And of course in the face of all this, Sandberg and the other women are right to demur. For the longest time, women have been expected to forfeit their identities in the blowtorch of motherhood, to have a baby and watch it subsume everything they have achieved over decades of professional effort. They are expected to drop down to three days a week, miss promotions, lose income, while their husbands surge ahead and get a free kid on the side. This imbalance makes me so angry that when I see male friends with young babies being praised to the skies for doing a fraction of the child care, I wish I were heterosexual purely for the satisfaction of having a child alone, rather than with a man who, however dedicated in theory to the 50/50 child care / housework division, will almost certainly end up taking the piss out of me.

But hang on. Even in this, I am being disingenuous. As I wander around the Facebook campus, stinging slightly from Sandberg's remark that the most important decision a woman has to make is the one about whom she has kids with—for all my ravings about men doing less of the child care, I know if I had a baby I would want to do everything for it myself. That's how my mother did it, that's how I want to do it and even if I was in a conventional marriage, I imagine I'd consider any baby I gave birth to as being more mine than his. I know a lot of women who feel this way and it gives their husbands a yawning great get-out, not to mention making them feel horribly excluded.

Meanwhile, the instinct of professional women not to discuss their domestic arrangements is understandable, but raises problems of its own. Now, not only are we supposed to feel guilty about if, when and how we have kids, but once we've had them, we're supposed to feel guilty about admitting they matter. Don't let on that it's difficult. Don't let motherhood interfere with your corporate persona. It's a fear that can bring on a weird fanaticism: choosing—for those few who have the luxury of choice—to take only two weeks of maternity leave or to travel during the late stages of pregnancy, gestures designed to shuck off the yoke of maternity, but that always strike me as the feminist equivalent of the preacher who, to illustrate his faith, goads poisonous snakes into biting him at the pulpit. It's the impulse behind all those slummy mummy columns that appeared in the British press ten years ago; the rash of "I'm a terrible mother" pieces, listing the gin and tonics, the sloppy housekeeping, the hilarious scrapes of the unmonitored children as if they constituted the most outrageous rebellion on the part of the women, but which ended up defining them in terms of their domestic arrangements as firmly as any 1950s housewife.

After the interview, I buy L's baby a branded sweatshirt at the Facebook gift shop and wander for a little longer around the campus. I walk past the graffiti wall, the fire pits, the soft play areas; the posters on the walls urging staff to be their "best selves" or asking them "What would you do if you weren't afraid?" (Hold a negative opinion about Facebook, perhaps.) Past the refrigerators stocked with energy drinks and the countless concession stands that give Facebook its fundamental character—as a place where you are never farther than ten yards from an opportunity to eat a free burrito. Eventually, I leave the campus and sit outside on a bench in the sun waiting for a cab. I sometimes think I could write an entire book about all the places I have sat waiting in the course of my job. Every railway intersection in the north of England; the convention center toilets of every major city in North America; the fringes of public gatherings in support of fox hunting / protesting the Iraq War / celebrating the queen's eightieth birthday / mourning the queen mother's death. Corridors, so many corridors. I can summon whole years of my twenties by envisaging the green patterned carpet of the Dorchester Hotel. It would be called *On Waiting* and would be described on the dust jacket as a meditation on the value of liminal spaces, and Alain de Botton, among others, would praise it to the skies.

The taxi comes. It's like all California taxis, stinking of old cigarette smoke and with ripped seats and a driver telling me the story of how he came to America from Armenia. It's considered bad form for journalists to quote what the taxi driver says, a barometer of how little interaction we have with "real people" outside the bubble, which is fair, and yet there is still something about these transitional moments. I often have a clearer memory of them than of the destination itself. Looking out of the car window, I feel alone, weightless, off the grid. I will wait, as we all wait, for things to pick up or to slow down, for my options to widen or dwindle. I will wait to be lucky, or unlucky. That evening, I fly back to New York from California and when I finally get to Brooklyn it is past midnight. The next morning, the bleeding has stopped and for the hell of it and because I can't think of what else to do, I buy a pregnancy kit from the pharmacy.

"Something very weird has happened," I say to L on the phone. I am standing in the bathroom, looking down at the spatula with its crosshatched blue lines. "I'm pregnant."

NINE

Falling

JOY AT THE CLINIC. Joy unconfined. It feels like winning a race. I have done it! I am the most brilliant person alive! Having decided that failing to conceive is none of my fault, I now accept full credit for the pregnancy. "You did it!" exclaims a nurse, rushing down the corridor to greet me, her colleagues hard on her heels. "We're so happy for you! After coming in here every week for so long!" (This is a stretch, even for me. I've been trying only for four months; what on earth do they say to women who've been going for years?) Dr. B is more cautious. "This is good, very good," he says, glancing at the results from my blood test, "but early days." He looks up abruptly. "Congratulations."

So here it is, the longed-for state. And how does it feel? It feels divine. I feel excessively, abundantly, ferociously pregnant. I feel as if I have done something unique in human history, not least because, overlooking the small issue of medical science, I have done it completely alone. A day after the blood test, on a warm morning in late March that either genuinely presages spring or feels that way as a side effect of my mania, I wander around Central Park, inhaling the sweet air and communing furiously with the cells in my uterus. I imagine myself apprising the baby of its dramatic eleventh-hour coming into being—how it clung on for sheer life during the deluge; how sure I was all was lost and then, hallelujah, you were there all along! Barely a week since conception and already it has a great story to tell.

"Oh, wow," says L, and if there is anxiety in her voice, I choose not to hear it. "Congratulations." And then, because she has been here herself, she advises me not to tell anyone, advice that I promptly ignore.

"I knew you'd do it!" says Merope on the phone from London, confirming my suspicion that this is not a biological event but a referendum on my character.

"A December birth," I say to Oliver, looking at the calendar and calculating a due date between my own birthday, at the end of November, and my mother's on December 16. "Sagittarius. The best sign."

"You're ridiculous," he says.

I don't call my dad, the person who will hurt most in the event of my own injury, which suggests that some part of my cautious self is still functioning. Neither am I so far gone as to believe the fizzing in my uterus is anything but imaginary, nor that its source is "human" in any meaningful way. Three days after conception, it is very much a "baby" in the same way that the synthetic meat in a fish stick is "crab." The only reason I know it exists is because fertility treatment has made me privy to an earlier stage of my pregnancy than nature intended, confirming the faint line on the pregnancy test long before a missed period. There is a good, evolutionary reason for this delay, shielding women who lose a pregnancy this early from the realization that they were ever pregnant. With fertility treatment, there is no such thing as not realizing anything; everything is realized, and recorded, and broken down into a thousand tiny cliff-hangers, every day bringing another blood test and phone call confirming or confounding the course of my pregnancy. I am pregnant on Thursday, but will I still be pregnant on Friday? And Saturday? I feel like a large ship trying to navigate my way down a narrow canal, or a creature scuttling over hot sand, trying to keep its points of contact with the earth to a minimum. Meanwhile, just out of reach, the promise of open water.

"Not good news," says Dr. B on the phone the next morning. I am standing at my office window, looking at the woman in the apartment across the street. She is doing yoga, as she does every morning. Bend and stretch; bend and stretch.

"Your hormone levels are dropping," he says, aiming for sympathy but sounding vaguely annoyed. "We'll do another test tomorrow, but if the numbers don't come up . . ."

They don't come up. The hormone, human chorionic gonadotropin, or HCG for short, is supposed to double every couple of days to indicate a developing embryo. Instead, it is steadily falling. I go on the Internet and type in "falling HCG numbers + still pregnant" and for ten minutes torture myself by reading posts from women with friends, or friends of friends, whose successful pregnancies defied the falling numbers.

It is hard for me now to revisit that moment, not because it was devastating, but because, in my memory at least, it wasn't. It was a flat, sad experience that left me more baffled than crushed. I simply couldn't make sense of it. A week earlier, I had confronted the possibility of never being able to conceive, and getting pregnant was clearly a reward for my suffering. That made sense to me. But a woman bleeds, gives up hope, gets pregnant, then turns out not to be pregnant at all? What kind of an ending is that?

Much later, a friend refers to this episode as "your miscarriage," and that is the real moment of shock, not from any delayed reaction, but from the implication that losing a pregnancy falls into a single category of experience. Going in week after week is traumatic. Putting everything on hold for a pregnancy that might never happen is traumatic. This five-minute pregnancy, which is, at least, a respite from the monotony of another month of no news, is relatively bearable and to equate its loss with that of women mourning a baby whose ultrasound photo has been on her fridge for four months, or who has already felt its first kicks, just won't do. To call this the loss of a baby is to sail very close to the right-to-life nonsense that anthropomorphizes a handful of cells. This is a disappointment, but it isn't a miscarriage.

When I go in for the official verdict a few days later, Dr. B is cheerful. "It didn't work out, but this is good news!" he says. "It means things are working, right? A met B."

I suspect that turning on one's fertility doctor is a stage of this process as conventional as standing up to one's therapist and I refuse to be cheered by his cheer. Goddamnit, what was I thinking? Letting this man pump me so full of drugs that my nascent baby got washed away in the flood? Why did I ever trust him in the first place? It's not as if I weren't warned about ob-gyns. If every profession has a section that is known to be nuts—in journalism, obviously, it's war correspondents, who can't sleep without the sound of bombs dropping; in orchestras, it's the brass section, specifically, the trumpet players (don't EVER go out with a trumpet player, says my friend Kate, a professional viola player)—

in medicine, contrary to the layman's assumption that it's the surgeons who are crazy, those godlike creatures who get their kicks from plunging their hands into other people's entrails, doctor friends say this is not in fact true. The maddest, baddest, most lunatic doctors—the ones you should never under any circumstances date—are the ob-gyns. It makes sense, if you think about it. Surgeons only save lives; obstetricians and reproductive endocrinologists can reasonably lay claim to creating it.

In this light, Dr. B doesn't look like my sane, affable, pragmatic ally, a man doing his best to get a result without bankrupting me, but a towering megalomaniac for whom no risk is too great. As he draws up a drug schedule for the forthcoming month's treatment, I snap, "I want to take fewer this time." I have no medical authority on which to base this request, but it seems to me intuitively right to assume that I lost all that blood and ultimately the pregnancy as a result of taking too many drugs. Dr. B raises his eyebrows and delivers a speech about fertility treatment being a blunt instrument, an exercise in risk and reward.

"Still," I say.

"I understand." But he gives me an exasperated look as if to say, "Do you want this to work or don't you?"

I do. I want it to work. But I have also, suddenly, had enough. The relief of having been pregnant, even for a day, brings on a motivational collapse the way that going on vacation after working too hard often unleashes the floodgates to illness. I've had enough of eight a.m. appointments and blood tests and ultrasounds; of tiptoeing around my own body as if it might explode in my face. I'm sick of banter with the nurses and game face with the doctor and of handing over my credit card after each visit, for the ultimate addition of insult to injury. I've had enough of pluckily pretending it's all going fine. I need a break.

"Take a month off," says Dr. B, genially. "Give yourself time to recover." The following weekend, a friend is having a birthday party in London and I decide then and there I will go.

"Perfect," he says and suggests I take my prescription with me; I can buy the fertility drugs more cheaply in England. I try to imagine handing over a prescription written by a New York doctor to the pharmacist in my dad's Chiswick branch of Boots and burst out laughing.

"They'll honor it," says Dr. B.

"They absolutely won't," I say, adding stiffly, "That's not how the NHS works." I think of the universal £8.05 proscription charge for all drugs in England and feel a surge of love for the motherland.

"Well, then," says Dr. B. He lowers his voice. "There are various Web sites. . . . It's called the gray market."

I haven't encountered this before: the shipping of drugs across state and country lines to exploit regional price differences. That afternoon, I go online and find small pharmacies in, for example, Scottsdale, Arizona, or San Antonio, Texas, undercutting New York suppliers by several hundred dollars, and that's before I look into Canada or Mexico. In each case, these Web sites inform me, I am required to scan my prescription and, with what feels like a big wink, e-mail it to the pharmacist before the drugs will be released. It's not a safeguard I can see the New York State Board of Pharmacy being impressed with if something goes wrong and I turn to them for redress. On the other hand, the drugs are up to a third cheaper. For an hour, I click on banner sales ads promising the "cheapest fertility drugs on the Internet" and try to convince myself that just because the phrase "savings of up to 40% on fertility medication bundles!" makes the pharmacy sound like a cash-for-gold pawnbroker, doesn't automatically mean it'll kill me. If there is one thing this experience has taught me, it is not to confuse my distaste for the sales pitch with distaste for the service being sold.

"Hmmm," says L. "I wouldn't." She is making the baby dinner in her kitchen. I am leaning against the counter, looking out across the Upper West Side toward Central Park and beyond. It's a view from a postcard, a skyline that will always be thrilling to someone from a low-rise city like London and that makes me wonder why I'm ever nostalgic for home.

"Did you tell him you want to take fewer drugs this month?" says L.

"Yes."

"But you have to really tell him."

"I did."

"No, you didn't."

"I DID."

L is as taken aback as I am that things aren't going smoothly, not because she's an optimist—quite the opposite; she tends toward alarmism—but because my role, generally, is to breeze along being untouched by things while hers is to see the potential for disaster in everything. Unlike me, L has no social qualms about being seen to be difficult, and not in the performative sense. There's a type of professional New Yorker who sends food back in restaurants and yells at cab drivers and won't go to Brooklyn because it's "too far" and hates the countryside on principle, and this person, inevitably, comes from Florida and moved to New York at the age of twenty-four. L, who really is from New York, sends back food and is always yelling at cab drivers, and hates Brooklyn, and will tell a doctor of thirty years' standing that he's going about things all wrong, but she doesn't think she is being cute while doing any of this. She doesn't think she is being anything. She is simply being, without repression or filter, and I can only look on from the sidelines in wonder.

"It's only been, what, four months?" she says. "You're panicking too early."

"Maybe I *should* just move up to IVF?"

"I don't think you need to. I think they messed up this month and next month will be better. But you have to be in control."

I infer criticism in this remark and bridle. The thing is, I don't really want to be in control, not over things I know nothing about. I don't want to be more active in dictating my treatment schedule based on—good god—intuition and an hour's research on the Internet. On reflection, I also don't want to buy cut-price drugs from Arizona. There are some things in life one knows not to buy cheap, eye surgery and sushi being the most obvious two, and to that list I now add fertility drugs. Even if the pharmacies don't try to palm off dodgy or out-of-date drugs on their mail-order customers, the way online groceries do with stale bread, the thought of injecting a substance into my body that has come via mail order—that has, over the course of its shipment, been handled by a chain of couriers, some of whom potentially work for Delta—makes my veins freeze in terror. I'd rather pay the full whack and have someone local to sue if I end up cooking my ovaries.

What I do know, with what feels like a mathematical certainty, is that the emotional cost of trying to get pregnant has to be balanced out with an input of joy. At the end of the week, I fly to London. For once the low English sky doesn't depress me but feels comforting, like a mottled old duvet thrown over my head, and when I walk into my friend's party on Saturday night, it is to faces I have known for twenty years.

"Are you all right, my little love?" says Merope, in a tone that, after almost two decades of friendship, instinctively avoids my dislike of certain forms of sympathy and makes her one of the few people to whom I would ever reply no.

"I am."

And for the space of the evening, I am. The party is in a garden, under a tent, where there are fairy lights strung across the canopy and a dance floor laid out on the lawn. I get giddy on cocktails and tell a friend of a friend, a woman I like but don't know well, how crazy my last month has been and she tells me her own fertility history, how, to her immense surprise, she conceived spontaneously with her husband in her midforties and how lucky that was.

"You'll be lucky, too," she says.

"It's a slog."

She smiles. "But it's so *interesting*."

From this vantage point, my life in New York looks unreal, a small, bright pinpoint on the horizon that disappears the minute I leave. London is the reality and New York is the dream. Even my failure to get pregnant dwindles to an abstraction—oh, that—and for the space of an evening I shove it off to one side. I know this impression is misleading, and that if I acted on it and moved back to London, the novelty of being home would wear off in five minutes and I'd be whining, once again, about my life having dwindled to a tiny set of known variables. But for one night, it is glorious. There are champagne and speeches and dancing. More old friends arrive and there are ecstatic hellos followed, hours later, by sloppy good-byes. Someone topples backward into a hedge. "Is she all right to drive?" "Oh, I expect it'll be fine." At the end of the night, there is the quintessential London experience: waiting for a minicab in a persistent light rain in clothes slightly too thin for the weather.

The next morning, my dad drives me to Heathrow. It has been a short visit, so he parks and comes into the terminal.

"This all sounds a bit brutal," he says, over coffee and bacon sandwiches.

"It is a bit." There is a long pause.

"Don't overdo it."

We don't say any more than this. My dad pays the bill and walks me to the security line. "KBO," he says, giving me a hug. "Keep buggering on." There are times when I really do love being English.

IT IS DIFFERENT this time.

"How do you feel?" says Dr. B.

"I feel messed with."

For five days, I have been injecting myself with a preloaded injector pen—same hormones, different delivery system—which, either because I've become cavalier with the needle or because something in the technology has failed, has bruised me terribly. The skin of my abdomen looks like seventies wallpaper, all bright purple flowers with a greeny-blue border. I feel altered, inert, hideously bad tempered.

"I can't sit on the subway for an entire hour to come and see you," I say to L on the phone after work.

"OK."

"It's a whole hour."

"OK."

"A WHOLE HOUR."

"OK!"

I tell myself it's chemical and will pass, like PMS or the low spirits brought on by a hangover. But it doesn't. "We don't know what these drugs are doing to us, in the long term," says a friend one day in a studio in Chelsea. She is coordinating a photo shoot with a supermodel I'm due to interview afterward. It's a job I might have turned down, if I didn't have one eye on the fertility meter and another two-thousand-dollar bill for drugs this month. I hadn't known about my friend's history of IVF.

This is what happens when you have fertility treatment; it's is like being the victim of a crime or getting a dog—suddenly everyone's a dog person or has a granny who was recently mugged. In this case, my friend's failure to conceive after two cycles left her with a negative view of the whole industry. Long before exhausting her treatment options, she had the strength of mind to pull the plug and eventually she and her wife adopted. She urges me to consider doing the same and although I make conciliatory noises, I know I won't do it, not yet. The threat of future ill health is too vague compared with the immediate threat of not having a baby. Will injecting fertility drugs turn out to have been unwise? Maybe. Would I trade in the possibility of having children to eliminate that risk? No. Every day, bigger risks are taken for much smaller rewards. After all, people still smoke.

A week after finishing the injections, I return to the clinic, where there are bowls of salad and trays of baked ziti laid out in reception. "Help yourself," says the receptionist and explains they have been sent over as a gift by a drug company. Next to the food, a sign has gone up advising patients that the clinic is being considered for a reality TV show and anyone interested should make themselves known.

"What's this?" I say. The receptionist shrugs.

"Really?" I say to Dr. B when I enter his office. "A reality TV show?" He raises his eyebrows. "What?"

"Bit intrusive, maybe."

He makes a dismissive sound. "Do you think those people on *Jersey Shore* regret doing it? They're all millionaires now." He looks at my charts, tells me to stop taking the drugs and ten days later I go in for the insemination. Number five.

"Whoa," says the nurse doing the preliminary ultrasound. "You have a lot going on in there."

I look at the screen; a lot of shapeless dark patches connected by strings.

"They look like spider's eggs," I say and shudder.

I have, once again, overreacted to the hormones. But Dr. B says not to worry; not all of them are mature. He makes a halfhearted gesture to indicate that, of course, if I want to be a purist I can call off the cycle and once again I say go ahead. He is in a good mood that day and after the insemination pulls up a chair. "What's been going, what's the news, what's happening in the world?"

"Beyoncé."

"Oh, yes, the nurses have been talking about that all week." Beyoncé's sister and JAY-Z had been involved in a fracas in an elevator, footage of which had been leaked to TMZ.

"What else?"

"Jill Abramson's been fired from the *Times*." I am curious to see what Dr. B does with this; his response to current events isn't always predictable. I once referred, in passing, to a famous female media tycoon, eliciting the rather surprising remark "She's a pure opportunist—the kind of person who'd have conspired with the Nazis. You know?"

Dr. B takes the news about Abramson and runs with it in the direction that the *New York Times* is an establishment stooge propping up the corrupt economic order. Something about quantitative easing and how we should have a gold currency. I get in a remark about pay disparity between men and women, which makes the young nurse at the desk look up sharply.

"Dr. B?" Another nurse puts her head around the door. We have chatted pleasantly for twenty minutes, the atmosphere as unstressful as the previous month's had been harried. Feeling grateful to the doctor, I get up to leave.

"How many eggs were there?" L asks, over dinner that night.

"Fewer than last time."

"What, four?"

"Something like that."

"Not more than four?"

"I don't think so."

She looks at me suspiciously. "Because if it was more than four you should've told him to cancel. Remember what happened last time."

"It wasn't. It was around four."

The weekend is lovely. The sun comes out and L and I take a walk along the Hudson with the baby in the stroller. I feel Zen in the face of all possible outcomes. On Monday night, I go into my kitchen and crack an egg against the side of a saucepan for dinner. Two bright yellow yolks slide down into the pan. I have never seen such a thing before and, standing at the stove, stare down at the eggs feeling bad for the hen. I am so surprised I say it out loud: "Twins."

I KNOW WHAT L is thinking: that if I go ahead with the insemination with more than a handful of eggs, I am risking not only my own welfare but hers, too. We are supposed to have one child apiece, that's the plan, a Venn diagram of two independent families, each with its own space and autonomy but that overlap in the middle for support. Two things threaten this vision: if I fail to get pregnant, or if I get pregnant with more than one baby. I can see her point; it would upset the whole balance of things. It would use me up, seal me into my own experience, make it much harder for our lives to converge. And while it would crucify me emotionally, financially, physically, even socially, it would also, obscurely, mean I had "won." This is very, very bad but every time I think of having more than one baby, my horror is mitigated by an imaginary air punch, the female equivalent of a testosterone high.

Anyway, I'm not having more than one baby because I'm not having any babies at all. What I seem to be having is another adverse reaction to the drugs. The Monday after the insemination, I look like I've had a large lunch. Two days after that, the swelling has spread to my sides. On Thursday night, I wake up in my bed in the early hours of the morning to the sensation I am drowning *on the inside.* The water level is halfway up my rib cage and rising. I drag myself to the toilet, throw up for a solid ten minutes and crawl back to bed ready to dial 911. Then I remember I am wearing huge black knickers with holes in the elastic and think, OK, give it five minutes.

"Oh my god," says the nurse when I go in on Friday morning. I am lying on the gurney and she is staring, horrified, at my bloated lower half. "You poor thing."

"Is this normal?"

"It happens."

"Nobody warned me."

That's not quite true. I remember Dr. B mentioning it, way back before my first round of injections, in the same way drug companies reel off side effects at the end of a commercial, the shortness-of-breath-paralysis-increased-risk-of-certain-types-of-cancer-seizures-and-in-some-cases-death spiel, and which I took with the same level of seriousness. In Britain, it's illegal to advertise prescription drugs on TV, and whenever I see a U.S. commercial urging consumers to ask their doctor about a particular drug, my baseline British credulity kicks in. Surely, I think, if the drug did any of those horrible things, the authorities wouldn't let them equate the experience of taking it with a couple having the time of their life on a beach? Surely no one actually *gets* those side effects?

Well, apparently they do, and I am one of them. Ovarian hyperstimulation syndrome (OHSS) is an overreaction to the fertility drugs in which the ovaries respond abnormally to an excess of hormones in the drugs and leak fluid into the abdomen. It is very common, says the nurse; about 35 percent of women taking injectable drugs get a mild form of OHSS and experience slight weight gain. In more severe cases, sufferers have to go into the hospital to be drained, and technically it can cause a blood clot and kill you. She carries on eyeing my lower half. "This is . . . quite bad," she says, but doesn't think I'm in any immediate danger. Awkwardly, I get up off the gurney and lumber to the subway, walking as if a horse has lately bolted from under me.

"What are you *wearing*?" says L that night, catching sight of me sideways on.

"What do you mean?"

"Look." I turn to look at myself in the full-length mirror propped up by her bedroom door.

"That is *insane*." I am so big-to-bursting that it appears, through the thin material of my leggings, as if I were wearing a codpiece.

"How's your fat pussy?" she says the following morning.

"Stop it. You know I hate that word." (I do, I hate it. It's a word for men who hate women and the women who love them—a great book title, by the way, for anyone who wants it.)

"OK." A minute later she says, "But how is it? Your fat pussy?"

Later that day, I return to my apartment and log on to my computer to find an e-mail from my friend Leila. "Hiya luv. How's your fat vag? I'm sorry but that will never, ever not be funny."

. . .

YOU CAN'T GET this fat on drugs alone. In all likelihood, the addition of pregnancy hormones has put even more pressure on my ovaries
and before I go in for a blood test I know I am probably pregnant. I
don't see this as cause for celebration. Gloomily, I think that I lost the
first pregnancy due to blood loss brought on by taking too many drugs
and will lose this, the second, due to the extraordinary land mass of my
midsection, brought on by taking too many drugs. I buy three over-the-
counter pregnancy kits and all three are negative. Still the bloating continues.

"Congratulations," says Dr. B on the phone a few days later. I am in
the deli buying Gatorade, one of the few things said to bring down the
swelling but which, after drinking gallons of the stuff, has succeeded
only in making my teeth ache.

"I'm a genius!" I say halfheartedly. "Or, you're a genius. One of
the two."

"It's early days," he says sternly.

"I know. I remember last time."

I don't bask in the news. I don't walk around Central Park communing joyfully with the cells in my uterus. I don't even work out the
due date and what its star sign might be. Instead, I trudge around my
apartment feeling as if I were wearing a space suit, waiting for the pregnancy to fail. Sure enough, a few days later, I go in for an ultrasound
and as the nurse moves the wand over my belly she hesitates for long
enough to telegraph bad news.

"I think I see more than one egg sac," she says eventually.

"What?"

She carries on squinting at the screen.

"How many?" I say. She holds up two fingers.

"Shit."

I look at the screen. For once, I can see what she's talking about, two dark dots orbited by light.

"You can see multiples this early?" I say.

"Yeah." She smiles. "I'm like the multiples whisperer."

Ten minutes later, as I'm handing over my credit card at reception, another nurse sidles up to me, eyes wide. "You know Sophia says she sees two?!" she says.

"Yeah. How's her form?"

"Pretty good."

If this had happened any earlier on in the process, I assume I would have freaked out. As it is, I can regard it only as a painful variant on the loss of a single baby this month.

"WHAT?" says L, who is not in that place. "Oh, no!"

"It's probably just a shadow on the ultrasound."

"That's not good," says L.

"I know."

And I do know, intellectually. All the risks associated with pregnancy increase when you're carrying more than one baby. Rates of miscarriage, preeclampsia and gestational diabetes go up. Placental abruption, when the placenta separates from the lining of the womb, is more likely to occur. The fetal death rate remains relatively small—1.6 percent of twins and 2.7 percent of triplets are stillborn, compared with 1 percent of single pregnancies—but the babies are more likely to be born prematurely, increasing the risk of cerebral palsy and other birth defects. Given the risk factors, this is why the conception of multiples is so frowned upon by public health bodies. In the last thirty years, both the United States and the UK have experienced sharp rises in the numbers of multiple births—a 75 percent increase in the United States, and 56 percent in the UK—largely as a result of IVF. (This surge is now mostly accounted for by twin births, triple pregnancies having declined in both countries thanks to steps being taken to avoid them.) But while the regulators in both countries acknowledge that this is not a good thing, the American Society for Reproductive Medicine allows that "in the United States, physicians and patients jointly decide how many embryos to transfer." In Britain, on the other hand, the patient is considered the last person on earth who should be asked how many embryos to transfer, because the answer is likely to be as many as are needed to bring this show to an end.

At the risk of belaboring the point, in the UK, public health policy is set so stridently against aiding the conception of multiples that, as a friend who'd had treatment back home put it to me, if you're under thirty-eight and having IVF in the UK, "you have to beg them to put more than half an egg back in." The Human Fertilisation and Embryology Authority, the industry's regulatory body, explicitly seeks to "reduce the proportion of multiple births after fertility treatment" and clinics are expected to come up with a "multiple births minimization strategy." No distinction is made here between the conception of twins and triplets; a multiple pregnancy of any kind is considered the biggest risk associated with assisted fertility and an overall bad business for mother and child.

I know all of this. And yet the only figure that concerns me is 27 percent: that is, the percentage of twin pregnancies that result in the miscarriage of at least one baby. My willingness to reassure L that, not only will the twins thing probably come to nothing but that I feel about it precisely as she does, is a false emphasis that makes me feel as shifty as one of those British bankers in the Far East who run up millions of dollars of debt and hide the receipts in their desk drawers until the entire economy is brought down. I don't want twins. Of course I don't. How could I? How would I begin to manage? It would be absurd, embarrassing. And yet the threat of losing them sets off a drumbeat in my brain that nothing I do will extinguish: *mine-mine-mine-mine.*

A few days later, I am having another blood test at the clinic when I hear a commotion in the corridor outside. The nurse excuses herself and a moment later I hear her colleague exclaim, "Mrs. X—triplets!" Then I hear what sounds like a high five.

"Someone's pregnant with triplets?" I say when she comes back in. She looks embarrassed.

"We're not supposed to say—but, yes." She beams. "After IVF. We put back two fertilized eggs and one split."

"That's terrible. What a nightmare." The nurse smiles at my naïveté, and for a moment I am jolted back to my pretreatment self. Of course. In a for-profit industry, one in which pregnancy is the only measure of success, high-order multiples start to look like the jackpot. Depending on how long she has been trying to get pregnant, the woman in question is probably half split between horror and helplessly declaring them hers.

Sure enough, twenty minutes later, while Sophia does the ultrasound, my clarity on this subject has flown out of the window and all I can think is how devastated I will be when it turns out one or both embryos has gone. Sophia peers at the screen. "You see? Two egg sacs," she says. She carries on peering. "Oh. Oh." Her face freezes. "OK, I'm not going to frighten you."

"What do you see?" There is a long pause.

"Be fairly confident you're frightening me. What do you see?"

"There's another small spot in the uterus, here." She peers some more and then comes briskly to her senses. "It's waaaay early. We're not going to panic. You can get dressed now."

As I'm getting dressed, another nurse comes in, picks up my chart and says "Oh!" Sophia shoots her a look. "It's waaaaaay early, so we're not going to panic her," she says.

Dr. B is away that week and it is his colleague, Dr. M, who takes the consultation. Dr. M is urbane, tanned, unrufflable. He looks like a man from a yacht commercial. My brain has gone into lockdown, working along the lines that if I don't get the information, the information doesn't exist. So I sit down in his office and say nothing.

Dr. M browses my notes with the mild interest of a man reading the racing papers. "Remind me how old you are?" he says.

"I'm thirty-eight. I'll be thirty-nine when I deliver—getting up there."

The doctor snorts. "Are you kidding? In New York, that's practically pediatrics." He carries on reading. "Your levels look good. They're consistent with a healthy single pregnancy or, at most, twins." He says this as if it were no big deal, the difference between, say, picking up one can of tuna at the supermarket or two.

"Twins," I repeat.

"It's quite common with IUI; a few more fertilize for insurance and never develop." The idea that I might be "getting away" with "at most" twins is too mad to fathom. "So I shouldn't panic?" I say meekly. Perhaps, after all, I have misunderstood. Dr. M walks me to the door.

"No!" He gives me a jovial pat on the shoulder. "Don't worry about this business of there being four in there. Let's see where we are this time next week!"

I am due to have lunch with Oliver that day and call him when I get into the street.

"Everything all right?" he says.

"Everything's fine. Although I should warn you I'm going to be ordering the onion rings *and* the cheese fries. I'm eating for five."

Oh, god. What on earth am I going to tell L?

YOU HAVE TO IMAGINE the worst-case scenario and work your way backward. This is Oliver's philosophy, an exercise in what he calls pessimism and I call optimism but that either way works on the assumption that by rehearsing the worst, one is able to neutralize its power. I am very good at rationalizing my fears, failing which, denying them, but Oliver is even better at this than I am. If there was a world championship in it—"Your friend learns she is pregnant, probably-with-twins-but-possibly-with-quads; you have five minutes to reframe her anxiety as a philosophically nonsensical position. Your time starts . . . NOW"—Oliver would win.

"One day you'll laugh about this," he says at the diner.

"I'm already laughing about it." As I say this, I can hear the slight ring of hysteria at the edge of my tone. "Can you imagine how much this is going to cost?" Not only does my insurance fail to cover fertility treatment, but the wording of the policy states that it doesn't cover "the side effects" of fertility treatment. "Do you think that includes having quadruplets?"

"I think it's too early to panic."

"That's what the nurse said. But there's nothing to panic about. I'm not having four. They'll have to get rid of—" Here I stop. How many—

one? Two? Three? There are, I know, doctors who believe whole-heartedly in abortion but have reservations about reducing multiple pregnancies and not only because it risks triggering a universal miscar-riage. The distinction between aborting a single fetus and aborting one of two, three or four makes no sense ethically, but there it is, raising the specter of a "missing" sibling and throwing weird light on the lottery element via which one embryo is destroyed and another is "allowed" to remain. As my friend Dan says to me a few days later, "What if you *are* pregnant with twins and you abort Einstein and keep Hitler?" ("You think I'm pregnant with Einstein and Hitler?" I say.)

I don't mention the possibility of quads to Dan. It is too shaming, too weird. Two are, depending on one's view, either bad luck or a gift from god. Four are straightforwardly a freak show.

"You could just go to England at the last minute and have them on the NHS," says Oliver, dragging a French fry through a puddle of ketchup.

"Yeah."

"Or the even-more-last-minute option."

"What?"

"BA flight crew. Trained to deliver babies, apparently."

"Good thinking."

"To fly, to serve."

I don't call L at work to tell her the news. I wait until that evening, when we're together at her apartment. Afterward, she is very quiet. The threat of quadruplets, even if the levels are more consistent with twins, is so insane, so hideous, that the only possible response is sympathy. I can sense her mind hovering like a cursor over the thing I have been think-ing all day: that this means I will almost certainly miscarry and have to start all over again.

On the phone the next morning, I tell my dad I'm pregnant without going into the details.

"Oh, love. Congratulations," he says.

"It's very early days," I say severely.

"Of course. So it's not multiples, then?!" My dad is well up on the lingo by now, but it is clear from his tone he is joking.

"Um, well, it might be two." There is a long silence. "But it's probably one."

"Wow."

To myself, I repeat, "It's probably one." To the few people I tell it might be two, I say "total nightmare!" because this is what I am expected to say. It is a nightmare. Single-mother-of-twins sounds like a cosmic joke, a punishment for the hubris of trying to cheat Mother Nature. But while I am shocked and appalled and terrified and the rest of it, there is a different beat still drumming away. In the quiet of my apartment and on the subway to L's, when I wake up and when I lie down at night: *mine-mine-mine*. It starts earlier than we know it, the body's defense of its own machinations, and way down deep in my bones I am cheering them on.

TEN

Rising

AS PROMISED BY DR. M, two of the four shadows on the ultrasound disappear inside of a week and it is confirmed that "only" two embryos remain.

"Two!" cries Dr. B, back from his holiday and leaping out of his chair as I come through the door. He holds up two fingers in a gesture of victory. "Two!"

It is hard to know, in this moment, what to panic about most: the prospect of losing them both, the prospect of having them both, or my doctor's maniacal joy. I smile censoriously.

"What's the matter?"

"I feel like a minority shareholder in my own body."

"Ah." He beams and points in the air. "But you have the deciding vote."

That night in L's apartment, I break the good news: that two of the four embryos have gone.

"So there's still two in there?" she says.

"Seem to be. For the time being. But, you know, it'll probably . . ."

"I'm going to have another one," she says abruptly.

"Good. Do."

"I will."

"You should."

It's not just that the balance between L and me will be upset if I have two. It's the discreet sense of one-upmanship between a woman with two children and a woman with one. We are rational people but we are not immune, L and I, to the cultural cues telling women that children are currency. I am pregnant with twins, ergo I have, in some sense, *done better* than if I were pregnant with a single baby, and from now on, every pregnancy ache, every complaint I make, will rest on the presumption of greater suffering.

Except, of course, that it won't because I am not going to have them. To be pregnant with twins when you're pushing forty and after months of fertility treatment is to live with the constant expectation that you will lose one or both. February 6 will not be their birthday. They will not be Aquarius. I will not have to move house and change lives and figure out how one person cares for two babies. L will not be forced to have another kid just to even things out. (Although, it does cross my mind that if I *do* have twins, and if she does try to have another baby, what if *she* then becomes pregnant with twins, making it three to my two and escalating an arms race that climaxes in our having nine kids between us and scoring the reality show of Dr. B's dreams?)

Over the next fortnight, the two blobs on the ultrasound take on stable identities, Baby A and Baby B. The former is cramped into the basement, the latter stretched out up top. Carrying two babies dilutes some of the obsessiveness of early pregnancy. It's a less intimate state, a gang instead of a couple. Rather than mooning over "my baby," I have the impression of two friendly strangers hanging out in my uterus, each doing his or her own thing (dividing cells) while I do mine (shoving handfuls of spinach into everything I eat and trying to avoid sudden movement). I run to the toilet ten times a day to check for the onset of miscarriage; whenever I sneeze or bend to pick something up, I agonize at the possibility that I've killed one of the babies. Every week, I wait for the ultrasound technician to tell me a heartbeat has gone. But the two blobs keep beating.

My friends receive the news with incredulity, then hilarity, as if I've come up with an ingenious new way to entertain us all. "I can't believe we were joking about twins and now it's happening," says Merope, on the phone from London.

"Sorry, I can't help laughing," says my friend Janice. "Imagining your face when they told you."

"You're going to look like one of those snakes that have swallowed a cow only standing on its end," says my friend Jake. "You will BURST."

"You're pregnant!" says my friend Selina. We are at a bar in Park Slope watching England play Italy in the World Cup.

"It's water retention," I say. And it is, mostly; I am still fat from the lingering effects of the OHSS.

She looks at me witchily. "No, it isn't." Selina and her husband have two children, both conceived spontaneously after umpteen failed cycles of IUI. When I tell her it's twins, she says, "Oh my god, I'll have one and I'm not even joking." Then she sobers up and shakes her head. "Brutal."

"It's only eight weeks. They might not stick." I say this apologetically. My pride in my superpregnancy is cut with equal parts shame. To paraphrase Wilde, to become a single mother of one child is unfortunate; to become a single mother of twins may be regarded as carelessness. I feel like the walking punch line to a joke, an illustration of the maxim "Be careful what you wish for." I am also laboring under the delusion that the more casual I am about the pregnancy, the less likely I am to lose it. Selina's superstitious machinery works differently from mine, however, and she looks horrified. "Why would you even say that?"

Over the next few weeks, I wait for the idea of carrying twins to normalize, but it doesn't. For minutes at a time I forget that I'm pregnant, then remember with the force of the original shock. What are they *doing* in there, these two people? Banging up against each other like bumper cars? Conspiring against me? For L, meanwhile, dismay slowly gives way to the satisfaction of telling me what to do. Pregnancy is a condition in which she is more expert than I and she throws herself wholeheartedly into the role of project manager, buying me vitamins and reeling off banned foods. When I fly to L.A. for work, she makes me promise to tell the TSA agent I'm pregnant and ask for a pat-down instead of the X-ray machine. (I do this on the way out, the words "I'm pregnant" sounding outrageous to my ears, but on the way back I'm too embarrassed and go through the machine as normal, then spend five hours on the plane worrying that I've radiated my passengers.)

The benefits of being ministered to by someone who has been pregnant herself are hard to overstate. I have watched friends go through pregnancies and spend half of the nine months reassuring their husbands that their input is priceless and that everything will be OK. By contrast, L's care is calm and practical and not predicated on the idea of pregnancy as an unfathomable experience. She isn't in a state of panic or awe at the idea of giving birth, nor does she need reassurance that her support is worthwhile. Her help is divested of reciprocal need, partly because she believes, as a matter of course, that she knows what's best for other people, and partly because, having had a baby already, she understands in ways I do not just how vastly I am about to need her—far more than she needs to be needed.

She is also uninterested in indulging the routine discomforts of early pregnancy. You might think a female partner would be more, not less, sympathetic to the aches and pains of pregnancy, but that is not my experience, and every afternoon, when I lie down in abject exhaustion, L rings me from work and is completely unmoved. On the weekend, she lies beside me and glances at my still-flat belly. "Hi, Baby A," she says softly. "Hi, Baby B."

Others are less sanguine. One day in May, I have lunch with an old friend I haven't seen for a while. I know he'll be shocked by news of my pregnancy and he is.

"Oh my god," he says.

"Yeah, so."

"Wow. Congratulations."

"Thanks!"

"I'm not being funny but: who's the father?"

I am generally quite even tempered, but when I'm not, the turnaround time between calm and Incredible Hulk is regrettably short. "Are you fucking kidding?" I say. "Who do you think the father is? What do you think—that L and I fell apart and I went out and randomly shagged someone? Who's the father? For fuck sake. There is no fucking father."

Then I feel bad and pick up the check. It takes twenty minutes for him to pluck up the courage to ask another question. "How's that going to work?" he says.

And there it is, the question we've been avoiding since L's pregnancy. If I have these babies, how will we arrange things? What will the babies be to L and what will she be to them? The answer is only partly to be found in the relationship I have with her baby. There is no honorific to describe what I am to him, no list of responsibilities or duties, and there is no word for what he is to me. He is not the price I have to pay for my relationship, but neither is he my child or my stepchild. He is at the center of us, the miracle over whom we both marvel, but I have no moral, financial or legal responsibility for him. Neither do I perform many of the most basic parental duties. I don't change his diaper, make his lunch, take him to the doctor or even babysit much, partly because L, still in the first flush of maternal anxiety, prefers to do everything for him herself and partly because she prefers to do everything herself.

I have always known this lopsided arrangement would be tolerable only as an interim stage until I had a baby of my own. What I hadn't anticipated are the ways in which its limitations would also prove to be strengths. There is something Kate, my best-friend-from-college, once said about godparenthood—that it should cater to the needs of the child not the adult. It makes no sense, she suggested, that when we have kids, most of us dole out godparent status to our best friends, establishing the role as one in which the godparent's primary relationship is with the child's parents. Surely it would be better for the child to have an adult in her life who wasn't a parent but whom she might consider to be exclusively "hers"? I think about this a lot in the early days of my pregnancy. In the year since his birth, my relationship with the baby has evolved to be oddly free-floating from my relationship with L. He is my friend, my buddy, a child in whom I have no stake other than love. That it's a love I'm not bound, by law or biology, to feel makes it all the more precious.

On the other hand. What am I doing potentially bringing two further children into a situation it takes almost half a page to explain? I can just about rationalize to myself why a woman without a child (me) might want to maintain a degree of separation from a partner with a child (L), given the vast difference in lifestyle between women with and without children. But two women in separate households with babies of a similar age who hang out on the evenings and weekends? If we're not a blended family then what on earth are we? If I have the babies and move apartments but remain living in Brooklyn, can we be said to be anything to each other at all?

The fact that I'm even considering this—moving within Brooklyn to be nearer Oliver and my friends rather than closer to L in Manhattan— is less a function of my doubts about the relationship than a vestige of my social obedience, a sense of what I am "allowed" and not allowed to do. Clearly, at this point, the proper course of action would be either to give up this nonsense of separate households, separate children and lobby to move in together, or else to do the decent thing and call it a day. There is no middle way, not even a word for it. Or perhaps there is a word for it and that word is selfish. It's selfish to carry on along parallel tracks, denying the children a second parent and creating two single-parent families. It's selfish, practically, morally, financially and environmentally, to maintain our independence while being together, like driving two cars to a single destination. And while my relationship with L's baby is full of sunlight and joy, how can it survive once I have my own children and am unable to travel back and forth to see him?

For the first time, I start seriously to question why I want to do this alone. It isn't just that L and I have conflicting ideas about parenting— very broadly, I am too mean in her eyes, and she isn't mean enough in mine—it's the historical weight each of us puts on those differences and our assumptions about where they might lead us. We both have a highly developed sense of self-preservation, for different reasons and expressing itself in different ways, except, perhaps, in this one mutual belief: that the way one protects children from harm is by controlling who is permitted to have access to them. I don't see a pedophile under every rock like my mother did (under every other rock, perhaps), but I do have a sense of unease about environment that I imagine falls outside the normal range. Have a baby with someone, split up, look on as the other person gets together with someone else, and before you know it, your child is spending large amounts of time with people over whom you have no power of veto. Or, have a baby with someone, *don't* split up, but fall out and raise them in the middle of a war zone. Or, have a baby with someone a long way from your country of origin and be effectively forbidden from moving home, because she doesn't want to move, or the courts won't allow it in the event of joint custody. The only thing more frightening to me than not having a baby is having a baby in a hostile environment.

It might seem strange to focus so relentlessly on the negative when, during the early days of my pregnancy, L and I have never been closer. And over the course of an average week, I go through many cycles of thinking this is good, we can do this, we can move toward something that makes more obvious sense. But a single sharp word and I am thrown back on my instincts: that, irrespective of whether I trust and love L, the only way to control for conflict around my kids is to have a front door to which only I have the key.

There is something I do when I'm feeling dysfunctional. I call my mother's family in South Africa. My aunt answers the phone—"Hold on. Hold on? Let me move my coffee"—and for forty-five minutes gives me a rundown of the family news, including the rumor that a seventy-year-old relative of ours has had a baby with a teenage prostitute, so that by the time we get round to my pregnancy, I feel like the most conventional woman alive.

"Twins, how wonderful," she says, not sounding remotely surprised.

My aunt has long given up on being astonished by life, but in any case, as one of eight children, with a paternal aunt who had twelve, and a grandmother who gave birth to seventeen, many of them twins, she has never doubted my ability to conceive.

"When are they due?" she says.

"February sixth."

"Aquarius. Good match with Sagittarius."

"They'll probably come early, though; twins do."

"As long as they're not born on January twenty-fifth."

"Why?"

My aunt laughs at the magnitude of what she is about to say. "Don't you know? That's my father's birthday." I yelp like a small dog being stepped on. My grandfather, the convicted murderer and child rapist, has been dead for sixty years, but I will move heaven and earth to avoid giving birth on his birthday.

My aunt's accent is broader than my mother's, but the inflections are the same, as is her undisguised happiness to have me on the phone. It doesn't matter what we say; to be talking to each other is reward enough. My mother's family was such a source of agony to her, so unresolved in its guilt and dysfunction, that it is only while talking to my aunt about my pregnancy that I realize how free I am from that pain. Without the example of my mother and her siblings' resilience, and without my own fury at the shame they were made to feel when they had done nothing wrong, I'm not sure I would have had the nerve to overcome my own shame and get pregnant. They survived the worst and came out of it wry, damaged, funny people, but loving, always loving, and if the babies I'm carrying ever come to fruition, they will have a stake in a history in which I feel only pride. As I say good-bye to my aunt, I experience a swell of emotion—not only toward her, but toward the idea of my children as descendants and heirs. There is nothing like new life to bind us more powerfully to what came before.

One warm Friday morning, I make my way up from Brooklyn to Manhattan for the last time. For the sake of nostalgia, I buy a bucket of coffee from Starbucks. I sit on the sofas beneath the framed pictures as the receptionist yells down the phone to someone who just got her period. The place looks very small and very ordinary, a small business run by people simply doing their best rather than what, at the height of my treatment, had seemed like an industrial machine. The doctors look different, too. Not so godlike; more like middle-aged men in white coats. In these, the early days of my pregnancy, when all I can feel is the roar of my own engine, I'm disinclined to give credit to the guy who jump-started the car.

Dr. B, it seems to me, is sensitive to this shift in dynamic and greets me with a wryness acknowledging that I no longer need him. Later, I write him a letter, thanking him for his kindness and expressing the profound hope that I never, ever have to see him again.

THE BOUNDARY for Advanced Maternal Age is thirty-five, which means that even if I wasn't pregnant with twins, I'd need a high-risk obstetrician. I am also being counseled by L, for whom all situations are, at some level, high risk. "You need to hurry up," she says, as I cast a reluctant eye, once again, in the direction of the doctor dating pool. "All the good ones go early."

This time at least, the selection is made easier by the fact that because my pregnancy will be covered by insurance, the vast majority of doctors can also reject me. Dr. K doesn't take my insurance. Dr. P doesn't take any insurance. Dr. F, who has a "good reputation" based on his Yelp reviews, operates out of a city hospital L says is staffed exclusively by hippies and gives new mothers a hard time if they have trouble breast-feeding. (This is the kind of thing she seems intuitively to know about the city, like how to order at Katz's and that the reason New York bagels are so good is "because of the water," which always gives me a pang for London, where I know things—where to catch the night bus; why you should never eat a hot dog from the cart in the street—too.) Dr. Y, the third doctor I call, does take my insurance but his secretary isn't sure she can find room on his list. He is an eminent high-risk ob-gyn, specializing in multiples and based at New York's number-one-ranked hospital, and I suddenly want him with the same passion I once wanted a limited-edition cardigan made by Missoni for Target. "Please. I won't be any trouble."

The hospital is on the east side of Manhattan, buttressed by the East River on one side and York Avenue on the other, a huge complex taking up an entire city block. The obstetrics department is on the ground floor, at the end of a corridor leading off a giant marble atrium. On the morning of my consultation, the waiting room is sparsely populated, mostly with other women on their own, a few accompanied by older women whom I take to be their mothers. On a TV fixed high on the wall, a commercial for a no-win, no-fee lawyer encourages users of a product called "vaginal mesh" to get in touch for a possible lawsuit.

Dr. Y has a large, kind face and a brusque manner I instinctively trust, but he appears close to retirement age and in the treatment room I brace myself for some cross-questioning about where these babies have come from. No such questioning occurs. There is no pastoral yammering, no chitchat to establish rapport. He doesn't ask who the dad is or why I'm at the consultation alone. He merely glances at my paperwork, says, "No IVF?" ("Just IUI," I say, preening), then tells me to lie down for the pelvic exam. I am delighted. If I want psychotherapy I'll pay for it. All I want from Dr. Y are two healthy babies.

I have been warned by a friend whose baby Dr. Y delivered that what comes next will be bad. But pain, like boredom, can't be imagined in advance, and even as the nurse looks down at me sympathetically, I assume my friend was playing it for laughs when she said that Dr. Y, while brilliant, has a quirk of physiognomy that in his line of work constitutes a serious drawback. Huge hands.

"You have a good pelvis," he says and for a moment I am too shocked to speak. My god. If this is how painful the examination is, what on earth will childbirth be like? I am suddenly flooded with gratitude to be pregnant with twins, for the increased chances it gives me of having a C-section.

"What are the characteristics of that?" I say eventually.

"Of what?"

"A great pelvis." Dr. Y frowns as if this were a piece of impertinence and says something about the distance between one bit of bone and another. Then he tells me my chances of a natural delivery are 50 percent. I get dressed and inform him that whatever happens, the babies can't be born on January 25. He smiles as if indulging a lunatic. "Guess what?" I say to L afterward. "I have a great pelvis!"

A week later, I start bleeding. It is slow at first, accompanied by cramps. "Call the doctor," says L but I don't dare; it is a Saturday morning and I have some unresolved Englishness about bothering doctors on the weekend. By Sunday, however, the bleeding is heavier. I lie down on L's bed, wrapped in cold dread, and will it to stop. Maybe I'll be lucky. Maybe one baby will survive. I get up and go to the bathroom, reeling with the realization that at some point over the past few months, the idea of losing one baby has become as devastating to me as that of losing the whole pregnancy. It is greedy to want these two babies so badly and yet, as I sit down on the toilet, I make a bunch of lightning-quick offerings as to what I'll give up for them both to survive: Anything. Everything. Health, wealth, ten years of my life. Complaining. Ingratitude. Fighting with L. Recreational whining about my job, which when it comes to it I really do love. I won't be afraid, or guilty or ambivalent about the future. If my babies survive, I will stop looking away and make plans. I'll be strong and brave and unapologetic. I'll live my best life. I cut myself off here as it becomes apparent that, at some level, I'm not appealing to god but to Oprah, and just then I feel something loosen and fall out of me. I reach down to catch it and, without looking, sense that in size and weight it is exactly as I imagine a four-month-old fetus might feel like. Sitting there, bloody hand between my knees, I burst into jagged sobs. L comes running down the hall.

"I can't look. I think it's a baby!"

"Let me see."

"I think it's a baby!"

"LET ME SEE!"

Looking away, I hold out my hand.

"Ew." She makes a retching sound. "It's not a baby." She carries on choking until eventually I look down.

"Ew." In my hand is what looks like a large and very bloody piece of uncooked liver. Abruptly, I stop crying.

Toward the end of my mother's illness my dad called me one Saturday to break some hard news. I was in the kitchen of my friend Suzanna's flat in north London and we were about to head out to lunch. The cancer had spread, said my dad, from my mother's lungs to her brain, and the doctor had just told them she had two months to live. I hung up the phone, crumpled into the wall and cried for thirty seconds. Then I snapped off the tears and said, "Let's go to lunch." Suz was at a loss. "Shouldn't we cancel?" she said. "No. I'm fine." And we enjoyed our day as if nothing had happened.

There are drawbacks to this approach. It doesn't generate vast reserves of sympathy for other people's tears. Neither does it make it easy to invite help from others. In the case of my mother's death, it probably prolonged the grieving process, because it meant that for a long time I persisted in the delusion that sadness will go away if you simply ignore it. In the end, I traveled to South Africa to see my mother's family and confront the sadness head-on, after which it slowly started to recede. But I still maintain that, in the first instance, the circuit break has its uses, allowing me to transition rapidly out of a state of panic and back to a semblance of normality, whence I can reassemble myself in relative privacy. Sitting on the toilet, I become eerily calm while L runs to the kitchen and comes back with a Ziploc. "Here, put it in here and take it to the doctor," she says. "And don't leave it in the fridge or Anita will eat it." (Anita: her son's babysitter, from whom no leftovers are safe.) Then she stands in the doorway and claps her hands to her face. "It's a baby! It's a baaaaby!" she wails. We both collapse into hysterical laughter.

Later, on the phone to the hospital, the on-call doctor tells me that unless I am in severe pain, I will have to ride it out and wait until Monday. Her voice is gentle and resigned and I realize she is trying to communicate a truth about miscarriage: that in most cases, there is nothing anyone can do. That afternoon, when L and I take her baby for a walk in the sunshine, I have a head rush that could almost be mistaken for joy—the thrill of confronting the possibility that the worst has come true, and that I am under no further obligation to fear it.

. . .

AS IT TURNS OUT, the bleeding isn't miscarriage. "It could be the result of dying fibroids," says the duty ob-gyn on Monday morning, after the ultrasound.

"Dying fibroids?" It sounds like a bad feminist rock band.

She shrugs. "We'll keep an eye on them, but they're nothing to worry about yet."

"Do you want to see the blood clot?" I lean over the side of the gurney and eagerly offer her the bloody Ziploc. "I have it here."

"Um." She frowns. "I think we're OK."

Over the course of the following weeks, I have several more false alarms, all of which end in unscheduled trips to the hospital and none of which turns out to be serious. Each time I go in, I drop another five hundred dollars on scans, with the result that just as my fear of miscarriage recedes, another fear pops up in its place: bankruptcy.

This is not an exaggeration. The maternity allowance provided by my insurers is capped at fifteen thousand dollars, a sum which, if you'd presented it to me before I got pregnant, I would probably have thought sounded generous. Now I know better. At the rate I'm going, I will have exhausted the pot long before the delivery. I could live in America for one hundred years and this would never get less shocking to me—the role played in life-or-death decisions by shortfalls in one's insurance, and the amount of time one is obliged to waste worrying about it. In my case, if either of my babies is born with one of the serious birth defects my insurers claim not to cover, I will have, somehow, to get us all back to England. In the meantime, I find myself nurturing the bizarre hope that when it comes to the birth, I will face something sufficiently life threatening to qualify for "emergency care"—triggering hundreds of thousands of extra funds in coverage—but not so severe as to kill me or the babies.

The costs are higher because it's a twin pregnancy, but after the initial panic, I never wish it wasn't twins—or rather, it's only once that I have a pang for how things might have been. This is a few weeks later on a work trip to Chicago, one of the last work trips I'll take, probably for years. I don't mind this. I've always been a grumpy traveler. I like having been places in retrospect and occasionally I have a good time while I'm there, but before a trip I tend to do everything I can to try to get out of it. I want to do this particular interview with a novelist in Chicago, however, not just because I need to earn as much money as possible before the babies arrive, but because it's where my cousin lives, the one who visited us all those years ago at my parents' house in Buckinghamshire and whom my mother counseled to have a baby by doing "whatever is necessary." Our mothers were only second cousins and never met, but I have seen photos and they looked startlingly alike. I would like to see Caroline, my closest relative in the United States, before the babies are born.

We meet in a French restaurant not far from the lake. Caroline took my mother's advice, married, had a baby and is now divorced and the single mother of a six-year-old girl. I watch them across the table. My cousin's daughter is much older-seeming than six. She reminds me of myself at that age—self-possessed, a little shy, basically forty—and the two of them together remind me of my mother and me. My cousin is solicitous without fussing and the bond is so strong you can almost see it shimmering across the table. Having one baby tends to be spoken of only in terms of deficit—like being a single mother—but that was not my experience and for a moment I envy them, the unique closeness of the mother to her only child. "Twins," says my cousin, a little enviously, too, then looks at her daughter, love of her life, and smiles back at me across the table.

When I get back to New York, it is to the first round of blood tests to check for fetal abnormalities. If I want, says the nurse, I can have a sex test, too.

"You bet."

"Your insurers might not cover it."

"How much is it?"

"Couple of hundred dollars."

I tell her to go ahead. I have never understood people wanting to be surprised by the sex, which seems to me like turning up at the airport not knowing if you are traveling to Iceland or Australia. A week later the hospital rings. The tests all look fine, says the nurse. "It's twins, right?"

"Yes." There is a pause.

"Two females."

"Oh, my word."

I am standing in my office and abruptly sit down in my chair. Two girls. So frozen have I been by the possibility of losing them, I haven't given much thought to what they actually are. Now I realize I've been suppressing a preference. "I wish you'd been twins with auburn hair," my mother would say, a reference to the red hair of her youth and her belief that the only way in which I could have been improved upon was if there'd been two of me. I loved her to tell me the story of the day the hospital rang with news that she was expecting a girl; of how she got off the phone and ran into the kitchen to tell my dad; of how, in her excitement, she chucked the last of the holiday champagne into the washing-up bowl, where she'd been washing the dishes before the phone rang. "It's a girl, it's a girl, it's a girl!"

Given the unpredictable nature of DNA, all babies are "random," but babies conceived the way mine were are particularly vulnerable to that charge. In the early days of my treatment, I had worried that having a baby via sperm donor might make that baby seem strange to me, the arbitrary result of a series of arbitrary choices. Now it feels as if everything in my life has led me to this. Every decision, every chance turn, every time I went out instead of staying in and stayed in instead of going out, was a step closer to this foregone conclusion. I have just spent twelve months making what felt like an endless stream of hard decisions, but now it seems to me that nothing about this pregnancy was a matter of choice. Of course I am pregnant with twins and of course they are female. How could it have been otherwise? The two strangers in my uterus disappear overnight. They are and always have been my girls.

L SAYS IT'S SIMPLE. I should move to Manhattan, somewhere within her neighborhood, so she can come round as often as possible. Oliver says, hang on. Maybe there's an argument for staying in Brooklyn, closer to a larger number of people with a smaller investment in me. And there is the third, nuclear option, which is to move back to London to be near my dad.

I'm not doing that last one. That would be insane. I love my dad dearly, but the idea of moving back to be near him, quite apart from the hassle, seems to belong to an earlier iteration of single motherhood, one in which the cost of having a baby alone is to give up one's adult life and effectively crawl back to the parental spare room. This seems particularly outdated in light of how old we all are when we start having our kids. If *we're* ancient, our parents are doubly so, and asking them to pick up the slack seems unfair. Besides which, for once, I would like to make a decision based not on the elimination of unpleasant alternatives but on something I actively desire. I just can't see what that is yet.

What I can see, as I enter my fifth month of pregnancy, is something I have not clearly seen until now. One parent, two babies. Not one parent, two abstractions, or one parent, two fetuses, but two actual babies, out in the world, who, as I know from L's experience, are going to scream and puke and need feeding approximately every two hours. This seems to me so lurid a proposition, so obviously absurd, that I can't believe it's actually legal. Why hasn't Dr. Y rung child services? Why isn't anyone shaking me and screaming "What the fuck have you done?!" What on earth did Dr. B think he was doing *congratulating* me for this outcome, let alone giving me the drugs to enable it in the first place?

More to the point, why has it taken me so long to clock how ludicrous this scenario is? For weeks, L has been hassling me about how I can't have two babies on my own and live in a walk-up and I have been snottily resisting her by pointing out that if an elevator building was a precondition of having a baby, the cities of Europe would be empty. Now I see she is right. What am I going to do—leave one baby in the street while I hoick the other one up the stoop to the apartment? How will I even get a double stroller up the stairs? I can order most of what I need for the babies online, but what if I miss the mail—how will I carry large boxes of diapers back from the post office when my hands are full pushing two babies? A door in my mind flies open and all the images I've been trying to avoid tumble out. Of being alone at three a.m. with a baby turning blue and no one to cry out to for help. Of trying to breastfeed two babies for months on end, slowly dying of loneliness and fatigue. All my ideas of self-reliance, of making a "positive" decision about where we might live, go out the window to be replaced with a single, desperate calculation: who, once the babies are born, can I anticipate getting more help from, the person who owes me because I helped her with her baby, or my oldest friend in New York?

If this calculation sounds unromantic, it is. Romance, the basis on which women have been making bad decisions for millennia, is not much of a factor here and I make no apology for it. Once you uncouple the becoming-a-mother part from the being-in-a-relationship part, romance is relegated to one of many considerations and not the most important, at that. I need help, I need love and I need a large degree of autonomy, although on that last one, I'm seriously starting to waver.

Only once, I think, does L raise a possibility that, in spite of my better judgment and hers, makes my heart leap at the idea of rescue.

"You could always move in here," she says.

It would be so much less frightening. It would be so much cheaper. I have no real sense of what it might be like to care for two newborns, so I don't even factor in the enormous benefit of a second pair of hands. Instead, I rehearse what cohabitation might actually look like. Slowly, my relief starts to wane. I imagine bringing the babies home to an apartment not designed for five people. I wonder what it would be like to have no space of my own. I worry about the implications of leaning too heavily on L, in a way that would make it infinitely harder, should it prove necessary, not to.

There is something else going on here, too, which I grope to define as having the courage to honor our relationship on its own terms. Marriage with children is the standard from which L and I might be said to fall short, and yet, in our case, it's merging households and becoming a "regular" family that feels to me like the failure. I don't want to make huge emotional decisions on the basis of cost, or to move in with someone because I'm either too afraid or too blinkered to imagine the alternative. The more I think about it, the more I realize that my fear of being alone with twin newborns is less acute than my fear of forcing L and me into something we're not. Children need clarity, and in a funny way, clarity is all L and I have. No blurred lines. No joint assets. No question of where do I stop and she begins. The line "I need space," like "It's not you, it's me," has become a euphemism for let's split up, but in our case it means what it says. It may be eccentric, and it lacks the most basic descriptors to reassure us it has a right to exist, but I'm finally starting to understand something about our relationship: that I like it fine as it is.

"I could," I say in response to her suggestion, and there is a long pause.

"Nah," we both say, in unison.

EARLY SUMMER is a good time to be pregnant. I'm not so heavy as to feel the heat as oppression, but I have a bigger surface area to soak up the sun. Standing on the street corner, waiting for the lights to change, I feel the warmth on my skin like a magnet drawing me upward. Things start to happen—not the eureka moment as to where I should live, but small, gratifying things. People give up their seats for me on the subway. (There is a definite social and racial pecking order to this. By far the quickest fellow passengers to offer me a seat are black men, followed by black women, followed by white women, followed by white men, particularly young ones in suits who tend to stare fixedly at their screens whenever someone old or pregnant hovers into view.) Strangers tell me how amazing I look and, in spite of my anxiety, I do feel amazing. I pity anyone who isn't pregnant or who isn't as pregnant as I am. For the first time in my life, I feel voluptuously, extravagantly female. Every time someone congratulates me, I hold up two fingers to indicate twins and

milk them for extra applause. People want to touch me, not just the reflex pat on the bump, but, as a friend who had twins noted, "They want
to touch you like lucky heather." When she was pregnant, a woman in
the street actually gave her a pound, "For the little ones."

"And you went straight to the bank and opened an account for them,
right?"

"No, I went and bought myself a latte on Broadway Market."

One day my friend Laura rings from London. "You're on the front
page of the *Daily Mail,* did you see?"

"No."

"I've just e-mailed you the link."

I open the page and read the headline. NHS To Fund Sperm Bank
For Lesbians: New Generation Of Fatherless Families To Be Paid For
By YOU. Britons are familiar with the identity of YOU, the notional
Daily Mail reader who spends his time trimming his hedge, setting fire
to pedophiles and fighting off illegal immigrants with a pitchfork, for
which Americans might substitute any fan of Fox News.

"That's brilliant!" I say. If offending the right-wing press was a national sport, my lifestyle just put me somewhere near the top of the medals
table, and Laura offers to send me a hard copy to frame for my wall.

"How are you anyway?" I ask.

"Fine. I'm going to a spa in Greece next week. It's the kind of place
where you don't speak and get pampered and come out the other end a
stand-up comedian or something. I rang my sister, by the way. She's
going to call you."

I hang up and a moment later the phone rings again. "Is that Emma
Brockes, soon to be mother of twins?" says Tessa. "Darling, did you see
the splash in the *Mail?* You're so on trend it isn't true. And it's so clever
of you to have two at once. You don't have to do all this over again!"

Talking to Tessa is reassuring until I remember that when she was pregnant alone, her mother moved into a house across the street and her sister lived ten minutes away. When L had her baby, she had a mother and a sister to drop by on rotation, on the days and nights when I wasn't there. I have my dad, who will be as wonderful and helpful as someone living three thousand miles away can be. But as I browse real estate Web sites that June, clicking on doorman buildings in Manhattan and boutique co-ops in Brooklyn, all I can see are small, overpriced cells of isolation. Every time I study a floor plan or think a lobby looks nice, I have a surge of hope that is instantly unseated by an image of me sitting alone at dusk, watching the door for someone who never comes. Even if I move to within a few streets of L, the demands of her life are such that realistically, she can be expected to look in only every few days. The same goes for Oliver and my other friends. This is the paradox of single parenting: it makes you more, not less, dependent on other people. It makes you think differently about your social networks and your place within them. Who can I lean on more like a brother than a friend? Who will still love me when I'm boring and unwashed and stressed out and exhausted and need more from them than I can ever repay? That last one is particularly shocking. Somewhere along the line, I realize, I am seriously going to have to ask other people for help.

One afternoon, L sends me an e-mail with a link to an apartment listing that is almost double the rent I am paying in Brooklyn. The floor plan looks familiar, as does the view from the window. Finally I glance at the address. It is in her building, the mirror image of her apartment, but one floor down.

"?!" I reply.

"!!"

I call her at work. "It's waaaaay too expensive," I say.

L takes umbrage at this, as if I were criticizing her apartment. "No, it isn't. It's actually not bad value for the neighborhood."

I take umbrage at this, as if I don't know the cost of things and that her neighborhood is so much ritzier than my own. "It's ridiculous," I say.

"Listen." It's always bad news when L starts a sentence with "Listen." "Listen," she says. "You need a service building."

"But do we want to live that close to each other? Isn't it weird?"

"I don't know."

I go to see it. The landlord is putting in new flooring and a new bathroom and most of the apartment is under polyethylene, but because it's an exact copy of L's, bar the fixtures and fittings, I don't have much trouble imagining it. It occurs to me, as I walk around, that he may not even want to rent to a single woman expecting two babies. But in any case, it's too expensive. Even if it's the kind of building I need, with a mailroom and an elevator and a maintenance team on site; even if it would be amazing to have L upstairs when I bring the babies home; even if the very fact that the listing came up in the first place, in a co-op that discourages rentals, is the kind of coincidence that feels like a gift from above—none of that matters because I can't afford it.

It is also, surely, nuts: to kind-of, sort-of live together but not. All my faith in being true to our version of togetherness collapses. It feels like a form of cheating, to have L's help and support and proximity-to-hand without the hard work of cohabitation. How would we explain it to the children? Or to ourselves? That we like each other sufficiently to be in daily contact, except on days when we don't? Assuming the arrangement held, what would the kids even *be* to each other? Not raised as siblings, but not stepsiblings, either. Cousins? Best friends? The victims of a half-assed piece of emotional evasion or beneficiaries of a radical new vision?

"Isn't it weird?" I say to Merope on the phone.

"It is weird, my little love, but you're forgetting you *are* quite weird."

My dad, who comes from a background in which people got married and stayed married until somebody died, believes, as he always does, that I am overthinking it. "Sounds like the perfect solution," he says.

"I can't afford it."

"Can you afford not to do it?"

For a second, I consider taking offense at this—yes, that's it, usher us toward a more conventional union so no one has to worry about my being alone—before I realize that the main person who wouldn't have to worry is me. L thinks I should take it, too, partly for loving reasons and partly, I suspect, because after our years of fighting over the merits of Manhattan versus Brooklyn, this would count as a decisive victory in her favor.

"It's not just the money," I say petulantly. "I don't want to live up there, it's boring. I hate the Upper West Side. I don't know anyone there. Who will I talk to?"

"You won't talk to anyone, you'll be looking after two babies."

Eventually, the landlord says other prospective tenants are interested and do I want it or not? Two steel front doors, a concrete floor and as much bureaucratic distance between us as between two complete strangers, and even then I'm not sure it's enough. And yet faced with the prospect of losing the deal, something unexpectedly rakes through my heart. I have no idea if it will work, or if it will expose the limitations of our relationship in a way that finally, decisively drives us apart. But until then, it feels like a life raft. Something else, too. We won't be living together, but we won't quite *not* be living together, either. For the first time, the outline of something surfaces that, during my endless agonizing about what we are or we aren't, I had never thought really applied: family.

YOU MIGHT WONDER at how "I can't afford it" changed overnight to "I'll take it" and the answer is fantasy math. This is something that, ordinarily, I deploy only to justify spending more than one hundred dollars on a single item of clothing, which is to say almost never. Now, after signing the lease and by drawing on every creative fiber of my being, I use it to rationalize an extra twenty-four thousand dollars on my annual rent bill. I'll cut my gym membership. I'll make my own sandwiches at lunchtime. I'll cancel HBO. I'll have my babies and never go out again; no booze, no dinners, no movies, no takeout. I'll wear my hair in a ponytail so I never have to get it cut and I'll go back to work the minute my body has healed. Obviously, I'll start spending my savings. If things get really tight, I'll sell my apartment in London, a measure that is 100 percent guaranteed to get me out of a hole, given the rock-solid dependability of the pound and the fact that I don't understand capital gains tax. Worst-case scenario—and this is the real psychological enabler of middle-class life—there is always the parental spare room.

All my doubts about the Upper West Side, meanwhile, dissolve in the head rush of having made a decision. "This the BEST result," I say to L. "Oh my god, I'm so happy."

"You're an idiot," she says.

I celebrate by doing something I haven't felt brave enough to do for almost a year. I used to enjoy going to meditation at Fiona's once a week, but while I was trying to conceive and in the early days of the pregnancy, it left me too frighteningly alone with my thoughts. On Tuesday night, a week before the move, I walk the two neighborhoods between my home and hers, where the two of us and our friend Daniella sit cross-legged on Fiona's bedroom floor, with the windows open and a summer storm rustling through the trees outside.

Thinking about the disjunct between my thoughts and my body— the trick of focusing on my breathing until it brings on a sense of my corporeal self as something distinct from the thing I call "me"—is something I usually find grimly unsettling. It gives me a feeling of how fragile life is, how easy it would be for the machinery to stop. Tonight it is different. In the first few moments of the session, a slew of terrifying words pop into my head—"amniocentesis," "bed rest," "labor"—but once I've swiped them away, I settle down comfortably into my body. I feel its heft, its solidity. The babies, who once seemed like alien invaders, now make sense of my body, their weight the physical manifestation of the joy that I feel. It used to be that whenever a woman over forty had a baby and wrote about it in the press, commenters would queue up to tell her that not only would she die before the baby grew up, but that she couldn't possibly identify with it when the age gap was so huge. As I sit there cross-legged, I have never felt so young and vigorous, as if I have five extra pints of blood flowing around my veins. I feel an animal-like power in my own physicality. I am ready to spring up, knock someone out, lift a house above my head. I am as young and strong and vigorous as my mother had seemed, in my youth, to me.

When the timer rings at the end of the session, we lie down on prayer cushions to talk about how it went. "I wasn't really into it," says Daniella. "I was daydreaming like I was at the bus stop."

"I felt like the oldest lady alive," says Fiona.

"I felt like an animal," I say and we adjourn to the kitchen for dinner.

Fiona, who is in her forties and single, is slight and pretty and, thanks to the success of her business, owns a large house in which she is embarrassed to live alone, and for which she is sure the contractors doing her refurbishment are judging her. Daniella is a fluent Mandarin speaker who used to cover China and the Far East for one of the big news agencies. She has one child and is forever being badgered by semistrangers as to when she'll have another. As we talk over dinner we all realize that looked at in outline, all three of us would be judged harshly by, as Fiona puts it, "people in villages."

"At least you have a husband," I say to Daniella. She makes a face. Not for much longer.

"Aren't you afraid of the overheads of doing it alone?" asks Fiona.

"I am. But I figure if nineteen-year-olds can do it, a nearly forty-year-old should be able to."

"You know," says Daniella thoughtfully, "sometimes you eat your own twin, in the womb."

"Really?" says Fiona.

"Yes. People who, like, have an extra finger, it's because they've eaten their own twin."

"How do we know if we ate our twin?" I say.

"We don't."

We consider this for a moment and then Daniella tells us about twin brothers she knows, John and Alan, both of whom had wanted to be doctors but only Alan succeeded. The dynamic between them was difficult, she says.

"John should've eaten Alan while he had the chance," says Fiona.

It is dark by the time I leave and I feel like a walk, so rather than taking a cab I stroll slowly back through the dark Brooklyn streets. Without a second parent, I want my children's lives to open up outward.

I want them to feel, through the example of the people around them, that our family is just one variable among many. I want them to know women who live alone, those who have kids and who don't. I want them to see that doing things differently entails not only an expense of will, but a degree of anxiety that, as long as you can sit around picking it over with friends, is a cost it is possible to bear. "It's all so interesting," my mother would say, of practically everything that crossed her path, even, in the end, of the chemo ward. Every week they wheeled over the IV machine and for three hours we sat there as the translucent liquid dripped down the tube into her veins. We speculated on the other patients. We poked mild fun at the do-gooders who crept around the ward handing out biscuits. "It's all so interesting," said my mother, with the slightest strain in her voice that only I heard. As a way of looking at things, it softened her passage through life, but that doesn't make it any less true.

AS A KIND of housewarming gift, L is resisting getting overly involved in my move and as a result, I do something stupid. One morning while I'm out, UPS dumps fifteen flat-packed boxes I have ordered from U-Haul on the sidewalk. L would, I know, tell me to go to the Turkish restaurant around the corner and offer the guy in the kitchen twenty dollars to come help me, the kind of thing she does very well and I do self-consciously and can't quite carry off. Gingerly, I pick up one of the boxes. It's heavy, and hugging it to my chest, I manage to wrestle it up one and a half flights of stairs before pausing to rest on the step. I see myself as if from the outside: fat, slow, overheated and alone, lugging heavy moving materials up two flights of stairs in defiance of everything I have read about miscarriage. I am being stupid and reckless and have pushed my self-reliance too far. And yet in that moment I feel close to elation.

I love moving. I love the sense that I am streamlining my life, editing it down to the bare essentials. I can't be stuck in one place if I'm *literally moving,* right? Literally moving while pregnant gives me, for those few days when everything I own is in seventy-five boxes, a sense of a life governed by order. My babies are in good hands because I'm finally jettisoning two thirds of my A-level notes and some gas bills from 2003. Everything I find makes me cry: old letters, photos, books, receipts, whatever random stuff made it over in the crates shipped from Britain. Even recent things reduce me to tears. Going through my fridge is like visiting a fertility graveyard. At the back is the half-finished packet of raspberry tea. Two open bottles of Gatorade stand in the door. In a black bag on the top shelf there are one thousand dollars' worth of leftover fertility drugs and an injector pen I am too superstitious to throw out. Finally, in the vegetable tray, I find a pulpy Ziploc smeared with brown liquid. I hold it up for a moment before realizing what it is. I am sentimental even about the blood clot.

I pack to music that night. Having my iPod on random play reminds me that the only time I've ever looked with envy on friends with younger parents was when they showed off intimate knowledge of the pop charts. Where their parents had Radio 1 on in the kitchen, we always had Radio 2, which was full of all sorts of horrors, but particularly on a Sunday evening when something called *Sing Something Simple* would come on, featuring a male voice choir and a man on an accordion and might as well have been called *Music to Die To*. My mother would get a dopey look on her face and say, "Songs from my youth," and even though I hated them at the time, they became songs from my youth, too. A single bar of this music affects L like a full moon on a werewolf, but it's too late for me, and as Vera Lynn's hits from the Second World War start playing, I curse my mother once again for conditioning me to like them. "There'll always be an England," warbles Vera, "While there's a country lane." I'm only thirty-eight, Mother; what did you do to me? After Vera pipes down, Sondheim comes on—*Sunday in the Park with George,* a musical I love, although I used to find the song "Children and Art" curiously soppy, a number that by Sondheim's standards is practically a crowd pleaser. I had always assumed that, when it really came down to it, Sondheim believed only in the "art" half of "Children and Art," and had thrown in the "children" bit to appease the out-of-town crowd. Then, a couple of years ago, I interviewed him. Toward the end of our meeting, I asked him what he'd have done differently had he come of age in a gay-friendly era. "Oh, I have no idea," he said brusquely, but a moment later he relented. "Wait a minute; yes, I do. I would love to have had children. And if I'd been one generation later, I would have."

After Sondheim, it's a quick slide through *Carousel, Annie,* the soundtrack to the TV adaptation of *Anne of Green Gables,* Petula Clark, Dana and Mary Hopkin, *South Pacific, My Fair Lady* (the Julie Andrews stage production) and *Cabaret* (the Judi Dench stage production) before I hit *Brigadoon.* People think *Brigadoon,* the 1954 musical starring Gene Kelly and Cyd Charisse as time-crossed lovers, is awful, but they are wrong. I once made Oliver sit through it and he spent a long time afterward trying to figure out the film's philosophical underpinnings; whether, as he put it, the town of Brigadoon, which appears through the Scottish mists once every hundred years, was being presented as a breach in the space/time continuum or merely as "a property of the observer"—an inquiry that goes a long way toward explaining why I love him.

"Brigadoon," sings the ghostly chorus, as I wrap plates and glassware late into the night. "Brigadooooon." I glance down at my belly, bumping up against the table like a mammal trying to push open a door. Hi, girls, I think. Welcome to the next eighteen years of your life.

ELEVEN

England

"WHEN ARE THEY DUE?" asks Jack a few nights later, during dinner at Dan's house. My friend Dan used to date women but now he is dating Jack and it's a great improvement. Jack is neither blond and stick-thin nor dull and unstable. He is funny and erudite and charming and cute. I think it annoys Dan how his friends keep going on about how much we love Jack, in the same way it used to annoy me when friends got overenthusiastic when I switched to women from men. Oh, all right, I would think irritably; be all bloody liberal and delighted for me. I sensed in their enthusiasm the implication that they had seen this coming before I did, and yet here I am, following Dan into the kitchen to hiss in his ear, "Jack's *wonderful,* I LOVE him."

Dan has cooked Jamie Oliver's roast chicken with rosemary potatoes and two vegetable dishes, plus a starter and dessert. I go back to the

living room, while Dan spends another twenty-five minutes on his and
Jack's cucumber mojitos.

"February," I reply, in answer to Jack's question, as Dan reemerges
and puts the drinks on the table.

"That makes them Pisces?" says Jack.

"Aquarius."

"Aquarius! Interesting. Tricky. What are you?"

"Sagittarius."

"Also tricky."

Jack thinks he might want kids one day but Dan isn't sure and
they're both curious to know how I made the decision. "It's so momen-
tous," says Jack. "How did you know?"

"I just knew," I say. This seems to me true when I say it. "I wanted
kids and it got so the idea of not having them became scarier than having them."

"But to do it alone," says Jack.

"She's not really alone," says Dan.

"I am," I say. I refuse to be cheated of the kudos of having no second
income or guaranteed help. "But I'm moving downstairs from L," I add.
"This week, in fact."

"Yeah, what *is* that?" says Jack.

It's two nights before moving and I have no idea how to answer.
Over the table during dinner I watch Dan and Jack. They are awkward,
as newish couples are, and occasionally superawkward, as are newish
couples in which one half only recently changed sexual proclivities.
There is a tense moment when Jack tries to tease Dan about a trip they're
taking in the fall. "I'm not paying for you!" he says archly, and I see Dan
bristle at the implication that he is the lady and Jack is the man. Regard-
ing L and me, I'm not the lady, I think, because I'm repressed and emo-

tionally evasive. L is not the lady, she thinks, because she can fix things and get lids off jars. I have never thought, about these babies, that I have to be "both" parents—male and female—because I have always assumed that whatever I am, I'm enough. But it's sad, I think, how no one wants to be the lady, not least because now that I am, by any definition, very much the lady, I have never felt more powerful.

On this particular question, however—"How will that work?"—I have no ready answer and shrug.

"What star sign are you?" I ask Jack.

"Pisces with Capricorn rising, which is why I'm not insane. I feel like my whole life has been an effort to check the Pisces in me." He sighs.

"Dan?" I ask.

"Libra," he says.

"Very straightforward," says Jack and takes a sip of his drink. "Isn't it lucky we have the science to explain all this?"

A WEEK LATER, I fly to London. It is the last trip I will take before the babies are born and I see a lot of people who hadn't known I was pregnant and most of whom, being English, have the good manners to wait until I've left the room to speculate on what my deal is. I run into my friend Jake in the office and as we head out to lunch, he stops to say hi to a colleague. As we walk away, he whispers, "She had a kid on her own but nobody's supposed to know."

"There should be a special handshake," I say.

A combination of the energy generated by the pregnancy and panic at my forthcoming financial doom means that for the first time in ages I'm in love with journalism again. A few days after my lunch with Jake, I do a job at an actor's house in a suburban street in north London, where I'm kept waiting for thirty minutes on the doorstep. It's raining slightly, a refreshing summer rain, and instead of being annoyed, I sit on a chair on the porch with my belly on my lap and have an almost plantlike feeling of contentment. I go down to Devon for a few days to interview a playwright and find everything charming, the spriggy hedgerows, the hot sun, the taxi charging through the close country lanes—even the overcrowded train on the way down, full of cheerfully drunk men in rugby shirts, which gives you an idea of just how out of my mind on hormones I am. I had caught the train in Oxford after spending a few days with Kate, my best-friend-from-college, who had come down from Birmingham to see me. "Baby A and Baby B," I said, introducing her to the lumps in my abdomen. She put a hand on each and burst out laughing.

"They look like two mice running under a carpet."

Being pregnant in England is different from being pregnant in the United States. Against the bone-deep familiarity of my old life, the journey seems greater, the outcome more amazing. I'm more sensitive to criticism, too. After eight years in New York, I can still look around and think, after all, what does any of this have to do with me? I can never tell from people's accents where they come from, and when they tell me, I never know what it means. At the guesthouse in Devon, by contrast, I take one look at the owner, a bluff man in late middle age, and am blinded by data, not just about the man—retired, from Surrey, of a type I can imagine enjoying putting a ship in a bottle—but about the assumptions he is almost certain to make about me. A pregnant woman traveling alone is a curiosity. A pregnant woman traveling alone for work is cause for mild excitement and against all my better instincts about chatty landlords, that evening, when I crunch up the gravel driveway after dinner at the pub, I pass him drinking sherry on the patio and accept his invitation to join him. "Twins and working, good for you," he says. "What does your husband do?"

The only surprising thing about this question is that I haven't been asked it before—that, and the fact that it still catches me off balance. There are so many potential answers: no husband, I'll be a single mother; no husband, I have a female partner; no husband, I have a female partner but we don't live together and we won't be coparenting; no husband, I have a female partner with whom I won't be coparenting but we are about to become neighbors so maybe she'll be a kind of aunt if that didn't sound so spinsterish?

"He works in finance," I say.

"Hmph," says the landlord approvingly.

I have a friend, Tiffany, a music journalist, who is a much better lesbian than I am—married, with a hyphenated surname she shares with her wife. As a matter of principle she never, ever lies about her life, except for this one time. Tiff was in Rome interviewing a rock star when a member of the publicity team asked her the same question the landlord asked me. Because Tiff had the measure of this woman, and because she was anxious about the interview and wanted to move on, she said, "He's a teacher." Her wife is, in fact, a teacher, but of course that's not the point, and when Tiff got back to New York, she felt so bad she confessed. When she told me this story weeks later, my first response was why on earth did you tell her? And second, why do you feel bad about withholding your life from some annoying PR? Tiff's wife, meanwhile, went up the wall and gave her a long lecture about cowardice.

I still don't know which of us was right. In the case of the landlord, I tell myself lying was a simple matter of expediency. He was drunk—to the point of giving me a lot of unsolicited life advice based on where he went wrong with his sons—and that made it imperative to end the conversation before he moved on to his marriage. I didn't owe him an account of myself, nor did I fear his disapproval—if anything, I could see he'd have gone the other way and been far too into it. Later that night, however, as I lie in the bed after removing the Union Jack throw cushions, my spirits sink. There's a certain shame in being unable to explain my situation succinctly, and while the landlord might not have disapproved, it would, I think, have replaced the impression he had of me as Super-Successful International Writer Lady with Woman Who Doesn't Know What She's Doing, or worse, Woman About Whom the Most Interesting Thing Is the Slightly Odd Way in Which She Had Children. This shouldn't have mattered. I wanted to be strong and brave and above caring what people thought, but equally, I didn't want to offer myself up as an object of titillating interest to a tipsy old man in a blazer.

This is how it goes, that night and in the following weeks, when I parry questions about my pregnancy with answers that veer wildly on the spectrum between truth, half-truth, lie by omission and outright falsehood. It's not that I want to lie, exactly. It's more that I don't have my story straight, not even when I tell it to myself, and in the coming years, I see friends in similar positions to mine repeat the same pattern— the journey from denial to defensive anger to that particularly British refuge "brittle cheer." One of these is a great, old friend with whom I meet up for dinner when I get back to London. She is single and trying to get pregnant via sperm donor and is still, by my reckoning, at the denial stage, whereas I am done with denial and elbow-deep in brittle cheer—with a few last vestiges of defensive anger in my system. That night at dinner, my friend tells me she has been to see a fertility consultant who has advised her that if she does manage to get pregnant, she should consider withholding the details from people, so she can pretend to have "shagged an ex" when asked about the father.

Over the cooling remains of my chicken tikka masala I am instantly, convulsively furious. Why, I ask, is shagging an ex seen to be the more respectable option? How is conning a man into having a kid he doesn't want, saddling both of you with a connection that will never, ever expire and visiting on the child a father who might or might not want to be involved with him, considered better than having a baby alone? For that matter, why is being married considered better than not being married? Surely it's just a question of taste? For god's sake, if you're that ashamed of what you're doing, you shouldn't be doing it. On and on I go.

"Wow, you're really angry," she says, taken aback. I return to my dinner, embarrassed.

It's not my friend I'm angry with. I'm not even angry with the fertility consultant. (Actually, that's not true. I think she's a louse.) I'm angry at my inability to give an account of myself that simultaneously (a) tells the truth, (b) avoids shame and (c) answers a casual questioner without inviting twenty-five thousand bug-eyed follow-up questions. There's no point in railing against that last one; the unfairness of one set of circumstances being considered neutral and another deviant or deficient is just how the world is, although for a while it is all I can focus on. I am a huge hypocrite, too, taking solace in the idea that my life is interesting, then shutting down anyone who shows any interest. In my head, meanwhile, I reply to anyone whose questions offend me with a loopy barrage of questions of my own. Like, while we're on the subject, how many times did you and your partner have sex before you conceived? Was it an accident? If one of you had turned out to be infertile, would the other have stuck around? Does it bother you that neither of your children looks like you or your partner? Does it make you love them less? Are you going to tell your child that his parents met on shag-bandit.com and somehow turned a one-night stand into a lifelong coparenting commitment? Or will you pretend you were "seeing each other" for six months before you conceived? How does your mother's undiagnosed mental illness affect your self-image as a parent? Is the twenty-year age gap between you and your partner in danger of stigmatizing your child at the school gate? Is your underpowered husband an adequate male role model for your children? To what extent do you think your children will be damaged by the fact that, in spite of both parents holding down demanding jobs, most of the domestic duties still fall on their mother? Is the fact that there's a nine-year age gap between your children a source of regret or indifference? Why was that, by the way? Was there a problem? What kind of problem? Whose problem was it, you or your partner's? How much did it cost to fix? If it wasn't for the children, do you think you would still be together?

The next morning, I call L from my dad's house. I don't want to tell her about my dinner explosion over shagging-an-ex. She gets quiet about these things, less demonstrably angry than me, but more anxious and upset. "How's it going?" she says cheerfully and I suddenly miss her with every fiber of my being.

"Great," I say. "But I'm ready to come home."

THERE IS ONE THING I have to do first. Tessa moved out of London to the home counties for similar reasons to those of my parents in the 1970s, which is to say the schools, the space and the countryside. Unlike my parents, however, she is a single mother with two kids conceived via sperm donor. No one is going to torch a cross on her lawn, but make no mistake, this was a brave move. Only once in its history has my home-town gone against the grain politically and that was in 1650, when Oli-ver Cromwell based his operations in the pub there, since when it has been solidly right wing. Almost everyone is white, almost everyone is married to someone of the opposite sex and almost everyone voted Con-servative in the 1997 general election, when the entire rest of the country voted for Tony Blair. There can be something expansive about small-town life—you can't avoid people the way you can in the city—and as-sumptions of bigotry can be unfair. On the other hand, Tessa isn't merely the town's sole single-mother-with-kids-conceived-via-sperm-donor, but the sole single mother at her kids' school, period. No one else is even divorced! In 2014! By the standards of the world in which I was raised, the way she—and I—have had our kids is sheer lunacy.

On a warm, dank day, my dad drives me out to see her, as either he or my mother would drive me around every weekend, to matches and swimming galas and the kinds of field-based fixtures I assume my city-raised children will never have. When we get there, my dad goes off to have a beer on his own in the pub and I buy some wine from the Tesco Metro opposite Tessa's house. From her doorstep, I can see down a leafy lane toward a park. When I was publicizing the book about my mother, Americans would ask me to describe where I grew up and I would say the nearest equivalent I had found in the United States was Darien, Connecticut. It always got a laugh, that line; I made "Darien, Connecti-cut" sound prissy and ludicrous, as a way of explaining how funny it was that my mother, of all people, had wound up in its UK equivalent, and to curry favor with an audience by owning my privilege. The thing I never said is how much the place meant to me. I might fondly disparage the conventional world I grew up in, but it contributed to the security that would, one day, enable my babies.

"Hello!" says Tessa, standing in the doorway, her two children peering out at her sides. "Remember I told you Emma was coming?" She ushers them outside, locks the door behind them and, walking four abreast, we make our way down the road to the park.

"Emma is pregnant with twins who were conceived the same way you were," she says to the kids. They look at me curiously.

"What are they going to be called?" says Alex, who is ten.

"I don't know," I say. "What do you think?"

"Charlotte and Nettie," he says firmly.

"What do you think?" I ask the six-year-old.

"Dustpan and brush," she says, giggling.

"Bucket and spade," says Alex and they run ahead laughing.

Tessa had her first baby alone when she was in her early thirties, a single heterosexual woman who assumed she would meet a man and settle down before the decade was out. (She didn't.) The reason she jumped the gun, she says, was that she had been diagnosed with polycystic ovaries and knew conceiving was going to be difficult. It seemed to her foolish to prioritize getting in a relationship over having kids, when having kids mattered to her more. A relationship could wait. Having children, with her health history, couldn't.

The first doctor she went to was in private practice in Harley Street and, she says, could barely disguise his disapproval. It was his receptionist who quietly recommended she go to one of the private wings of the big London hospitals and this was much better; they were professional and disinterested, although, in line with medical guidelines in the UK, they did make her go to see a counselor before committing to treatment. Tessa also saw a hypnotherapist who made her cry by asking "Isn't it selfish to want children?" then charged her £110.

There was no open market for sperm. Everything had to go through the hospital, which gave her a choice of three donors, about whom she was told almost nothing beyond what they did for a living. (She boggles at the amount of information I have been able to get about my donor, including how tall his parents are and what all his siblings do for a living.) Her first child was born after a single IVF attempt; the second took more than five years to conceive and the entire exercise set her back some fifty thousand pounds. Back then, the NHS wouldn't treat single women wanting a baby, but in any case, says Tessa, she doesn't believe the state should pick up the tab for what is essentially a lifestyle choice.

I'm not sure I agree. It's true that not having kids doesn't kill you and the NHS is broke and there will always be higher priorities. Still, limiting access to fertility treatment to rich people feels a little too much like social engineering. There is, of course, always adoption, or, as some people like to suggest casually, "Why don't you just adopt?" (These people, I notice, are rarely if ever adoptive parents. If they were, they would understand that there is no such thing as "just" adopting; the demands of the adoption process are as onerous if not more so than fertility treatment, and as fraught with difficult decisions. For example, would you adopt from abroad? If you are a white parent and there are no white babies in-country, would you adopt a baby of another race, even though many adult adoptees of transracial families are at best ambivalent about it? Would you adopt an older child? Would you go through an agency that put pressure on a teenage girl to have and then give up her baby rather than to have an abortion? If you went looking for a baby at an orphanage in China, what measures would you take to ensure the child's birth parents were actually dead and not merely too poor to look after him or her? If it turned out they *were* alive, would you consider writing them a check so they could take home their baby rather than simply moving on to the next child on the list? I don't have answers to any of these questions, but they are unavoidable for those seeking to adopt. And all of this is before you get to the fact that, if you are single or gay and living in large swaths of the United States, adoption can be ferociously difficult.)

One advantage of adoption is that formal advice given out on how to talk to the kids about it is based on lessons learned from generations of adoptive parents doing it "wrong." When Tessa's children were young, she says, there were no books on the subject of having kids via sperm donor, except a crap one featuring a hedgehog wearing flip-flops. She joined a donor-exchange network—an online support group made up of families similar to hers—which helped a bit, but mostly she made it up as she went along. I must make an involuntary face, because she says, "What?"

"Oh," I say. "Um. I can't imagine joining a support group."

"It was quite helpful," she says.

"Hmmm."

When her eldest asked where he came from, she told him Mummy had wanted a baby and the hospital had given her one. This held for a few years, until a friend had a stern word with her about lying. A fairy story about how babies were made—one that cut out the involvement of a man—just wouldn't do, so she changed the story and said, "Mummy wanted a baby and a nice man helped." To which her son inevitably replied, "Where is the nice man?"

Obviously, I say, I am going to have to come up with my own answers to these questions, although, assuming everything goes well with the birth, I figure I have five years on the clock to get my story straight.

"Hahahaha," says Tessa. "It starts MUCH earlier than five."

She pauses to call the children over from the swings, where they have been trying to push themselves high enough to go over the top.

"Mummy, Mummy, did you see?"

"I did, darling, don't go too high. Alex, how old were you when I told you how you were conceived?"

"Um. Four?" says Alex.

"Three?" says Jessie.

They run off again. Eventually, she says, when they were still very young, she gave up and answered every question truthfully, technical terms and all, then warned them not to tell anyone at school; not because the information was shameful, but because she didn't want them lording their knowledge of words like "sperm" and "penis" over other kids in the playground.

"And did they accept it, what you said?"

Up to a point, says Tessa. They were relaxed about where they came from, but they complained now and then about not having a dad, which made her feel very guilty. She looks at me curiously for a moment. "But you have someone on the scene, right?"

"Yeah, but we're not. I mean, it's entirely separate operations. She won't be their parent. Also, living together just doesn't . . . I mean, we'll see how it goes. I only have a year's lease on the apartment. I might not even stay in the U.S. Maybe I'll have the babies and want to move home." She stares at me.

"That would be a bit abrupt, wouldn't it?"

"I probably won't. But you know. I *could*."

"Right," says Tessa.

I identify more closely with Tessa than with women having children in couples, but still I'm belligerently uninterested in joining any of the support groups. The very words "support group" make my skin crawl. Why do I need support when there's nothing wrong with me? And what value is that support anyway? I don't have brain space for a bunch of untested orthodoxies from women potentially more neurotic than I am. It doesn't occur to me that it might simply be nice to talk to people who have been through similar things, or that the strength of my rejection is a throwback to a rickety old line of denial. If I am snobby about talking to women who have been in my position, then I must be snobby, at some level, about the position itself. I don't see this at the time. All I know, the day of visiting Tessa, is that I refuse to seek common cause with a bunch of women I know nothing about.

Tessa and I leave the park and saunter back to the house and while the children play video games in the lounge, she and I sit on the patio under a late-afternoon sky. We drink some wine and she tells me how difficult it is to be the only family in town that looks like hers.

"Come and live in New York among the lesbians," I suggest. "Your kids won't stand out at all."

"But I'm not gay!" wails Tessa. It always infuriated her when she went on holiday with her sister and they were mistaken for a couple. "This is my SISTER," she would say to anyone who glanced at them twice. "I sometimes wonder if we should have moved to Brighton," she says. But she didn't want to live in Brighton. She isn't remotely bohemian. She wants to live where she is living, where the children have space to run around and where, in ways more profound to her than the technicalities of how she got pregnant, she feels that she and the children belong.

"How was it?" says my dad on the way home.

"Good. Helpful. She's so nice." I look out of the window. "It's funny to be back here."

"Yes. It all seems like such a long time ago."

I look at the pubs and antique shops and feel a surge of affection for this part of the world, followed by a tremendous surge of smugness for not living here. How clever of me, I think, to be having these babies in New York, where they will not stand out in a crowd. How clever of me not to aspire to the conventional life that Tessa feels guilty for denying her children. Well done, me, and well done, L. We have beaten the system. We have budgeted for every eventuality. There is just one thing. As with so many of my assumptions of how things will be after the birth, I have overlooked a tiny detail. I can control where we live and I can control how we live and I can control who has rights to my children. But, oops, I forgot about this. I can't control whom they love.

TWELVE

New Year's Eve

IT'S NOT A FANCY BUILDING, in fact it's quite ugly, a utilitarian sixties block a stone's throw from the park. The apartments are large and airy by Manhattan standards and the views of the skyline are spectacular, but nothing about the block could be said to have "character." If I had, before now, been asked to describe my dream home, I would probably have gone for a nineteenth-century town house, with cornices and fireplaces and all that *Architectural Digest* junk. In a million years I wouldn't have imagined a midcentury American box, with standard-issue low ceilings and in a building with the kind of twenty-four-hour infrastructure—a front desk, mail room, large maintenance staff and management—I've always thought spoiled and intrusive. How little we know ourselves, even this far into life.

Within a few days of moving, something occurs to me: that I've been nervous in every place I have ever lived, starting with the house I grew up in—so many points of access, so quiet after dark—through my flat in north London, my dad's house in west London and finishing with the converted brownstone in Brooklyn from which I've just moved, and where the fire escape outside my window felt like an open invitation to burglars. Having a lit corridor outside my door rather than a dark street is instantly, miraculously curative. I stop lying awake at night listening for noises. I don't jump at the sound of the plumbing. L once told me that one of her favorite places to be was in her house growing up, with her parents and siblings vaguely around but none of whom was expressly bugging her. Now I discover this, too, the joy of being alone while surrounded by people.

And not just any people. Old people! "Oh my god, you must be so happy," says Merope when I tell her I have effectively moved into a retirement home. The building is designated by the city as something called a NORC, or a naturally occurring retirement community, which means that many of the residents bought their apartments for next to nothing when the building went up and are now in their eighties and nineties. As their apartments come on the market, families with young children move into the building, giving it an eccentric air of half old people's home, half day-care center, with games of chicken—walker versus stroller—playing out in the corridors daily. (The walkers have it every time.) "Welcome to the three of you!" says Pam, a friendly retiree, on the day I move in—when you are expecting twins on your own, people hear about you before they have seen you—and elsewhere on my floor there is a widow in her eighties, several other retired single women, a family with youngish children and two women roughly my age. Of the nine apartments on my floor, six are occupied by single women, a number that rises to seven after the family in the apartment next door moves out and yet another single woman moves in. "It will be so nice to have babies on our floor again," says Pam. For a few months, before the babies arrive, I have never felt so safe and secure.

I had half wondered whether, in those first weeks after moving, my living arrangement with L would be exposed as the ridiculous proposition it had so often seemed—that we would spend so much time in one or the other of our apartments that the vast expense and small inconvenience of living one floor apart would become increasingly hard to ignore. In fact, we enter a honeymoon period in which the loveliness of living almost together is nothing to the luxury of living sort of apart. Being in identical flats throws into relief a rainbow of domestic differences that hadn't been so apparent when I was living in Brooklyn. L cares less about mess than she cares about dirt. I don't care about dirt, but I care about mess. When I go upstairs, the toys and crayons scattered on her living floor leave me twitching with existential unease. When I return to my tidy-ish flat, I note the dust bunnies in the corners and the occasional bug in the sink and thank god L isn't here to protest. (If L sees a bug, she is up all night going the full Joan Crawford.) These might seem like trivial differences, but when you live in close quarters I don't think they are and I think they are only made worse by children. At least in the early days, having separate homes keeps us sane.

The act of leaving my flat and walking up one flight also imbues even daily visits with the tiny frisson of occasion. When one of us snaps, the other goes home without it being construed as a histrionic gesture. And while hanging out is much easier when neither of us faces an hour-long commute, to my surprise *not* hanging out becomes easier, too. It doesn't mean anything anymore. I don't sit around thinking, how often does one have to see someone to imply the relationship counts? Is three times a week enough? What does it mean if we decide not to spend the weekend together? There's no marriage or joint mortgage between us, nonetheless a commitment has been made: my twelve-month lease is unbreakable and this, too, is surprisingly reassuring. I have the long-overdue realization that relationships, like everything else, rely on a balance between independence and the right level of curtailment of freedom to liberate one from the burden of choice.

I go up for breakfast. L sometimes pops home between meetings and comes downstairs to stick her head round the door. We have keys to each other's apartments and don't bother knocking most of the time, because the locks are there if we need them. When L comes to mine, she heads straight for the fridge and browses for anything new and exciting. (It's a noble search, given its fruitlessness. In spite of Merope's best efforts to teach me to cook in my twenties, I still live mostly off pasta and sandwiches.) When I go to L's, I head straight for the remote because I'm too cheap to buy cable downstairs. At some point, we realize by looking at the available networks that we live close enough to share Wi-Fi.

"Do you want to?" I ask. "If I can figure out the airport extender?"

"Um."

"Yeah, me, neither."

In the evening, I go upstairs to eat with L and the baby, and then we hang out together watching TV. I'm usually quite tactile, but this far into my pregnancy my core temperature is molten and all I want is to lie diagonally across my own bed at night and find no one else there. We bid each other good night and I go home. And this feels remarkable, too.

One evening, L sits on the sofa with her son reading a book she recently ordered from Amazon. It's about different kinds of families. "'Some people have two mummies,'" she reads, pointing to an illustration of two badgers wearing earrings with a baby badger in their midst. "'Some people have two daddies. Some people have one mummy, some people have one daddy.'" Her baby, who isn't a baby anymore but a toddler and the most delightful child in the world, isn't quite old enough to formulate questions and we are off the hook for a little while yet. L and I exchange glances. "Some people have a neighbor," she says, sotto voce.

THIS PERIOD WON'T LAST. I know this. Before the babies are born, L and I have all the time in the world to flop around enjoying each other's company and marvel at the wonder of her son. My children will change things in ways neither of us can begin to imagine. I look down at my belly sometimes and boggle that a mere half inch of skin, fat and fluid stands between me and the rest of my life. Half an inch and three months. Overnight, I am suddenly huge. I look like a stick of asparagus stuck to the side of a watermelon. I feel immense, mighty. I stalk around town sheathed in black leggings, knee-high black boots and a brown cashmere cardigan, through which my belly protrudes like a torpedo. I'd thought the advanced pregnancy belly would feel wobbly, like a beer belly, but it's strong and firm and I'm so preoccupied with it—that and the need to eat all the time—that it becomes hard to concentrate on anything else. One morning, I go to the Waldorf for a breakfast interview with a nice English actress whom I can barely hear I'm so focused on forking as much bacon into my mouth as I can in forty-five minutes. When we get up to leave, I push back from the table and she says with some relief, "Oh, you're pregnant!" Listening to the tape afterward, all I can hear is her pleasant voice underscored by a faint and terrible gulping.

I put off all the things I'm supposed to be doing. I don't book a prenatal class. I don't buy a crib or a stroller. (Jesus, a "double stroller.") I'll inherit a lot of basic baby clothes from L, but I haven't figured out how I'll manage in those months after the birth. How does one person, even with help from upstairs, physically meet the demands of two newborns? "You need a baby nurse," says L, and although I know she's right, I don't start calling around or interviewing. I don't want to break the spell.

And I am busy in those last months of the year. My new rent burden hasn't started to bite yet and I'm sufficiently padded that it won't for some time—not until it is added to by the shocking, crippling cost of child care. But I see it coming and through the end of summer, into autumn and winter, I work frantically. I write endless columns. I spend months on the piece about the playwright in Devon, across multiple re-writes and late-night revisions. I tour some of New York's parks with the head of the parks department, as part of a series about world cities. We start up on 125th Street, in what used to be a rough neighborhood and is now full of ritzy grocery stores and hipster BBQ restaurants. I arrive early and, after buying a foot-long pastrami and Swiss sandwich from Subway, sit on a park bench and look out at the water. When my interviewee arrives, accompanied by a press attaché and several assis-tants in black SUVs, he gives me a history of the park and talks more generally about the need for clear sightlines in the city's green spaces. He is, he says, against low tree canopies because they obscure the view. "You'd be concerned as you turned a corner," he says vaguely, scrutiniz-ing the tree line in the distance, "because you don't know what's waiting for you."

WHAT SHUNTS ME ONWARD, in the end, is the fluttering. One night I get home from L's and peel off my leggings and boots. On the bed, I roll to one side, the only comfortable position left, and that's when I feel it; a fluttering from pelvis to ribs, as if tiny gills were brushing my insides. My scalp contracts. My god, these things are actually alive. I am woefully unprepared for this birth.

In the United States, as far as I can tell, there is no single central authority for educating pregnant women and, in my case, no stern reminder from my doctor to crack on and sign up for a prenatal class. No one has told me to do anything at all, and because I will never deprogram from the assumption that a patient should only ever act on her doctor's orders, I wonder if perhaps I don't have to. Maybe the birth is something I can turn up to at the last minute and, like any deadline, leave it to adrenaline to sort out. I've watched a few YouTube videos on how to breathe during labor. Women give birth in rice paddies, etc. Apart from those early scares with the blood, it's been an easy pregnancy—no morning sickness, no mood swings. My only unscheduled visit to the doctor over the summer was to Dr. Dolphin, my eye guy, for blocked tear ducts—take *that* to a therapist—so really, how hard can it be? Then up they start with the fluttering and all that flies out the window.

Here is (one of) the problems with the free market: it shifts the burden of responsibility onto the consumer. If I receive a bad service it's because I made the wrong choice and the choices in this case are dizzying. Some prenatal classes in New York come with lunch or a goody bag sponsored by a baby store. Some cost hundreds of dollars and entail the services of a "baby planner," or a "maternal wellness consultant," or, in my case, a "twin concierge," who will come around to frighten me in my own home. Some last an hour, some last a day, some are stretched out over two months. All I want is to be in ill-fitting yoga pants in a chilly church hall, being told what to do by the state. Instead, I have to decide between a brand consultant and someone who calls herself a "mompreneur."

There are other factors, too. The city may be more forgiving than a small English village, but even so, Manhattan is not exactly a place light on judgment and I have to be careful not to put myself in a situation where I'm going to feel freakish. A friend who is trying to get pregnant alone tells me of going to a class on how to manage the injections and discovering, too late, that everyone else there had come in a couple—some gay, some straight, but all of them in pairs. She'd been feeling quite chipper until then. But those three hours with no one else to hold the needle left her feeling self-conscious and lousy.

In the end, I choose a prenatal group for expectant mothers only—no partners allowed—which also slyly eliminates the need to worry over whether I should be attending with L. The class is in a posh neighborhood on the East Side, run out of the back of a boutique maternity store where even the nipple cream comes wrapped in three layers of tissue paper and the racks are full of things I don't want to think about: nursing bras the size of trampolines; breast pump paraphernalia that looks like you could smoke crack with it. As I ease myself down into a chair that first evening, the word "flange" floats unhappily in the corner of my eye.

There are twelve of us arranged in a circle around Claudette, the group leader, who tells us that she was a sales executive before the birth of her daughter, then ditched her corporate job to set up as a maternity guru. It's the kind of potted bio inclined to make me sneer my own face off, but before my snootiness can get off the ground, Claudette goes on to say that the parenting industry is running way out of control and we should take every piece of advice, even hers, with a pinch of salt. She advises de-subscribing from all but the most reliable pregnancy mailing lists and consulting our friends more than we consult the Internet. Above all, she says, we should let go of the idea we can anticipate every outcome. Ladies, know your limitations.

Claudette asks us to go around the circle and give three details about ourselves: our names, what hospital we are delivering at and when we are due, such a narrow data request I wonder what she is playing at, until the first woman says, "Hi, my name is Tara, I'm delivering at Lennox Hill. My husband is a lawyer and—"

Claudette laughs gently and holds up a hand. "Yeah, we don't do that," she says. "What your husband does for a living—I don't give a shit."

Boo-ya! I am still feeling great about this when she adds, "By the way, does anyone here *not* have a husband?" No one raises her hand and I hesitate for a second too long. "Only we have quite a few single moms in the other group." Now it is too late to say anything. Claudette, who doesn't know I am single, looks over at me and I feel myself redden; perhaps there is a big *F* on my forehead for Fatherless children. "And we have only one twin mom, right?" she says. The other women look over. I smile and do a coy little wave.

This isn't like concealing my life from the old man in Devon. There is no prurience here. No one is drunk and flirtatious. This is a maternity group in which it might be useful to seek advice for my particular circumstance. But if I fear the other women's judgment, it's for the very good reason that as I sit there, I am being horribly judgmental about them. There is the woman who turns up in flip-flops to indicate she lives on the block (i.e., she is incredibly wealthy and keen to show this fact off). There is the one who looks sixty years old—it can't be her egg, surely!—and comes in every week fully made up and in a lot of gold jewelry. For a couple of weeks, I think the one with wild hair and gum boots might be more on my wavelength, until I find out that her dog has a surname.

Half the group doesn't work and is treating pregnancy like a full-time job and of course, I am sniffy about this, too. They know which drugs they do and don't want, which is better, cutting or tearing, and how many hours into labor they want surgical intervention. (This is fine, says Claudette, as long as they don't alienate their doctors so monstrously it interferes with their care.) One woman asks how close to her delivery date she can carry on going to spin class. "Wait," says Claudette, looking down at her chart. "You're still going now?!"

I never come clean about my personal life and I never stop feeling it as a small, profound failure. Over the course of six weeks, however, something miraculous happens; our collective terror starts to eclipse our differences. Every week we sit in the circle, owl eyed and jittery, but less reserved with one another, and kinder. The rich lady in gold worries she doesn't have an adequate support network. A youngish woman by the standards of the group has only one month's maternity leave and doesn't know how she will cope. Claudette answers questions about overheated apartments and difficult mothers-in-law and anxious husbands, through which we learn a little of one another's lives, but not much, because once these issues have been dealt with, we are to a woman obsessively focused on the delivery. It's like kids at camp trading ghost stories after dark: someone knows someone who had to have multiple surgeries after her kid came out basically sideways. Someone knows someone who could never sit down again. The worst of the rumors emanate from Europe, where, the circle has heard, women are allowed to die rather than be offered the option of a C-section. Claudette tells us about a member of her downtown class who comes from Sweden, where, she says only half-jokingly, they let you stay in labor for five days and when you ask for a C-section say, "Give it another hour! You're nearly there!"

When I repeat this story to friends, it is with an expat superiority that implies I am tougher than these pampered Americans. When I meet an American at a party who tells me she recently gave birth—"I pushed for THREE HOURS before they jumped in and gave me a C-section!"—I nod sympathetically, while luxuriating in the thought, three hours?! Try three days, love, with only an aspirin and a cork to bite down on for comfort. I go on endlessly about how C-sections are overused in the United States—almost one in three births in 2013, compared with one in four in the UK and fewer than one in five in Sweden.

It's a pose. Even my masochism stops short of making me want to push out two babies and I've been away from Britain long enough to waver in my blanket defense of the way the NHS does things. I have a friend in London my age who gave birth to twins vaginally and without a lot of bother, but I know of others who were in labor for a hellish forty-six hours, denied a C-section for what they suspected were either ideological reasons or reasons of cost. And so, while I continue to recoil from women who insist on their right to a highly individualized set of birth goals based on a few hours Googling "episiotomy," when it really comes down to it, most of my chauvinism is for show. I will be thirty-nine when I deliver and as such I am weepingly, convulsively grateful to be in a country where the comfort of the mother comes first. (Actually, the preeminence of the mother's comfort is a bit of a myth about American childbirth. The consumer might be queen, but there's no question that C-section rates are high in the United States because they suit the hospitals. In New York, a surgical delivery can cost a patient's insurer fifty thousand dollars—something I panic about every time I think of it—but to the hospital, a twenty-minute C-section can cost a great deal less than having a woman clog up the delivery room for twelve hours. Apart from anything else, it allows more babies to be born in a day.)

I have no interest in the mystical experience of giving birth. My "birth goal" is for all of us to be alive at the end and for me somehow to wind up not bankrupt.

"DO YOU WANT ME to come with you?" says L. We are in her kitchen a few days before the amniocentesis, the procedure in which amniotic fluid is removed via a large syringe through the belly. It is supposed to be painful and traumatic, not only because it carries a small risk of miscarriage, but because the testing of the fluid for chromosomal disorders brings with it the threat of bad news.

"No," I say.

"OK," she says cheerfully. "Good luck. Call me when you're out."

Before the amniocentesis that fall, I had never seriously considered what a late-term abortion is for. I think at the back of my mind I'd imagined it was a safety net for scrappy teenagers who didn't know they were pregnant until six months in. It hadn't registered that it was primarily to prevent the birth of severely damaged babies. Neither had it occurred to me that when campaigners talk about restricting abortion to the first twelve weeks, they are condemning a woman to carry a baby to term, irrespective of problems that emerge only in late pregnancy.

The amnio, therefore, is a frightening proposition, the last opportunity to exit the pregnancy if something turns out to be wrong. Because of the small risk of miscarriage, some of the women in my prenatal group, particularly those who've had fertility treatment, say they aren't going to have one, but it was never a question for me. Of course I'd have an amnio, and of course I'd have a termination if either baby turned out to be damaged. These were the assumptions I held going in, rooted in my deepest convictions about a woman's right to abort. What I hadn't realized was how nineteen weeks pregnant would feel. They kick more in the evening and when I lie down. They go berserk when I eat a bowl of lo mein. Baby A moves in short, sharp bursts and Baby B is more languorous, as if she were doing a gentle backstroke across a pool. Sometimes they fight, the bottom one kicking in the direction of the top one, who responds with an evasive squirm. "Cut it out, Baby A," I say and am struck once again by the insanity of twins: two human beings having a brawl in my abdomen. Once a fortnight, their heartbeats thunder on the monitor. They are stupendously, thunderously alive.

A few weeks before the test, I am made to attend a genetic counseling session in Midtown, the only mandatory piece of pastoral care in the entire process from conception to pregnancy. After giving me the talk about Down syndrome, congenital heart defects and cerebral palsy, the counselor asks if I want the fluid gathered during the amnio to be put through a second layer of screening, at a cost of several thousand dollars.

I start to stutter, hopelessly. I had no idea there'd be an element of choice in all this. I know my insurance won't cover the extra tests. And while, during fertility treatment, I rationalized medical decisions partly on the basis of cost—forestalling IVF for the cheaper IUI—that felt different. The worst outcomes were financial and emotional. There was never any risk of material damage. In this case, if I deny myself an extra level of certainty for the sake of a few thousand dollars, I may give birth to a baby who is devastatingly ill, or whom, rightly or wrongly, I don't think I have the capacity to care for.

Or will I? The counselor explains that the second layer of testing looks for relatively obscure genetic defects, the severity of which, when detected in utero, might be impossible to judge. So I would potentially be aborting on the strength of a "maybe."

I drag myself home, having told her I'll call in a day with my final decision. I am livid at being put in this position. If I don't pay for the extra tests, will it make the delivery more frightening? What does it mean to factor in cost when the stakes are so high? Just how bad must the news be to consider terminating the pregnancy this late in the day? Trying to answer these questions gets me nowhere. What does, in the end, is a moment of clarity so overwhelming that I remember precisely where I was when I had it; in the hallway of my apartment, three steps from the bathroom.

This is how it is, I think, and how it will be for the rest of life once the babies are born. From that day on, "maybe" is the best I can hope for. Maybe they'll be OK and maybe they won't. The element of faith even the faithless among us are compelled to feel once our children leave us to walk through the world is the basic condition of parenthood. It is the thing that permits us to function alongside the knowledge that, at any moment in the day, something terrible might happen, not to us, but to them. In the absence of guarantees, all I can do is get used to it. I don't order the tests.

SO FAR, my experiences at the hospital have only been lovely and they change the way I relate to New York. When I first moved here, it sometimes felt like being twenty-two again and in my first job in Scotland, when I didn't know whom to ring or how anything worked. Six years later, I still have to grope to find the correct American word for "sockets" (outlets), and "loo paper" (bathroom tissue), but for a brief period, being part of the life of a grand institution makes the city feel fractionally more mine. It is satisfying to know where every exit of the hospital comes out, or to avoid the Sabbath elevator on Friday nights into Saturday, when it stops on every floor, or how to take a shortcut from Dr. Y's to the ultrasound department upstairs. This is where, one Thursday morning before the amnio, I turn up for the detailed anatomy scan, a painless if annoying exercise that can take more than an hour for twins, in which every limb and internal organ of the babies is measured. It requires both babies to be awake and stretched out, and if they don't cooperate, it means canceling and coming back another day.

On the bus journey, I listen to the latest episode of *Serial,* the podcast everyone is talking about that fall, but when I get to the waiting room, I take out my headphones and stare vacantly around. I occasionally feel sorry for the men with their wives in the waiting room. When appointments run late, I observe them stealing glances at their watches, only to look up into the furious faces of their spouses. Perhaps it's different when it's not your first baby, but my appointment could be hours late and I would be quite happy sitting there doing nothing. This, it seems to me, is one of the best things about pregnancy; there is no way of speeding it up.

"Emma?"

Her voice is sharp and I look up. I had noticed this particular nurse before; she is short and rotund and usually quite cross. She is very cross today. "Come on," she says irritably when I'm stretched out on the gurney, addressing my abdomen and looking up at the screen. Baby A has been a dream, but Baby B is asleep and won't stretch out. The nurse shakes the wand on my belly. "Unfurl your hand so I can measure it," she says. "Come on, baby!" She presses a button and the gurney tips my body, headfirst, in the direction of the floor. "This sometimes wakes them," says the nurse, and I feel the weight of the babies slide glutinously toward my ribs. On-screen, Baby B uncurls a single finger. "Come on!" snaps the nurse.

Eventually, the baby stretches out just enough to be measured and the nurse slides the wand over my belly. "She's keeping her legs closed," she says approvingly. "Daddy will be pleased."

I am so surprised by this remark, it takes me a moment to respond.

"Let's hope it stays that way," I say (what?!).

After we are done, I get dressed, go downstairs and call L on my way to the bus stop. "How'd it go?" she says.

"OK. I mean, she sexualized my twenty-week-old fetus. But apart from that, all good."

I can never get any work done when I've had a scan in the morning, and when I get home, I sit on the sofa and flip through a book I have ordered from England. It is by a stout NHS doctor (I have no evidence to suggest she is "stout," other than the slightly brisk march of her prose) and contains lots of information about how to care for a newborn. Her main piece of advice is that, until it becomes second nature, new mothers should keep a written record of when each baby feeds, sleeps and poops.

I just can't see how I will do it. Trying to figure out how to keep track of two babies feels like the infant care branch of string theory: a mind-boggling math problem along the lines of if Baby A is hungry at nine a.m. but hasn't pooped and Baby B poops at nine-thirty a.m. but isn't hungry, how high does their mother have to turn up the oven when she puts her head in it at half past eleven? For my birthday that year, I ask Oliver not to buy me a present but instead to read the first three chapters of the baby book and, using his giant brain, figure out a diagram for how I'm supposed to do all of this. "When to feed them and change them, and how to monitor it all," I say.

"It's hilarious that you're asking me this," says Oliver, "but I'll try." And he does. He reads the material and makes me a chart in Excel, to keep track of who's doing what—columns for when each baby poops, wees, eats and sleeps—and I stick it on the fridge door next to the ultrasound pictures and a drawing done by one of my friend Liese's six-year-old twins, a smudgy figure in crayon (me) with the words "Babies Are Coming" written ominously over the top. I quake every time I look at it.

I start to have stress dreams. I dream that Baby A, the lower of the two babies, shows up on the ultrasound with a lizard's tail, which I reach in to pull off and instead detach its whole arm. There it lies in my hand, bloody and white and as limp as a noodle, with tiny curled-over fingers.

"You need to stop fussing with it," says L flatly when I tell her about the dream.

"You think I should've let it keep the tail?"

"Yes." She is, in so many ways, more liberal than me.

L had told me the amnio doesn't hurt as much as people say but that I would be well advised not to look at the needle. On the morning of the test, I stand in front of my mirror at home and shiver at the thought of being stabbed—twice—not subcutaneously, as with the injections I performed on myself, but way down into the uterus. By the time the results come in, I will be two weeks shy of the New York state abortion limit, and if there's a decision to be made, there'll be no time to linger.

The doctor, whom I hadn't met before, is reassuringly businesslike, exuding vibes of this-is-100-percent-routine and telling me, "Most women say it's not as painful as they think it'll be." When he first entered the room, I thought I'd detected a tiny pause in his momentum when he registered I was alone, but if he did, he quickly recovered. It is the week before the Scottish referendum and, noticing my English accent, he says, "What are the Scots going to do—reinstate the Stuarts?"

"Very good!"

With twins, doctors inject blue ink into one of the amniotic sacs, to ensure they don't test the same baby twice, and, as promised, the first doesn't hurt. As he draws up the needle again, the doctor says, "This one is going to hurt more because of the baby's positioning. She's very low, near your bladder." A moment later I feel a white-hot stab of pain. Yowza. "OW," I say. Then, just as abruptly, the pain shuts off.

"That wasn't as bad as I thought!" I say, hysterical with relief.

"No higher praise," he says and sweeps out of the room.

At L's that night, I tell her about the doctor. "Young guy," I say. "Nice. Efficient. Probably quite junior." My first-choice doctor hadn't been approved by my insurers and, although this isn't how it works, I had assumed I'd been given someone cheaper. L, who has never received a piece of information she hasn't subjected to a thorough background check, looks him up.

"Oh my god," she says.

"What?"

"This guy—he's the head of the whole department." She keeps reading. "He's some kind of wunderkind."

"No way."

"Yeah. He goes to Congress to testify about raising the abortion limit. He's, like, the rock star of high-risk obstetrics." I have sometimes wondered if there is anything in this life that can't be turned into a competition, and here the answer comes, no. How I preen, from then on, about coming under the care of the most illustrious high-risk ob-gyn in Manhattan.

It is a peculiarity of the hospital that all test results are posted online to the patient's private mailbox, often days before a doctor rings them. This is supposed to increase transparency, but in reality, it just opens a quick and efficient route to paranoia, leaving the patient to interpret highly specialized medical data using Internet searches and guesswork. A few months into my pregnancy, I'd received a result that to my untutored eye had seemed to suggest I had a low lymphocyte count, which I'd Googled and within five minutes self-diagnosed cancer. And what to make of this, an assessment that went up a few days after the detailed anatomy scan: "The cervix could not be appropriately visualized by transabdominal exam and in some views appeared short"? I loved the idea of point of view in all this. "In some views, the cervix appeared short; other people, however, thought it looked beautiful."

The exceptions to this free flow of information are the results of the amnio, which are serious enough to skip straight to the phone call. A few days later, the genetic counselor rings. Everything in the test has come up fine. A week later, I run into the rock star doctor after a routine scan and we stop for a chat. "Ankles slim, all looking good," he says, casting a professional eye over me. Smiling, he moves off down the corridor. "Stay pregnant!" he calls over his shoulder.

AMONG ALL MY NIGHTMARE scenarios involving babies with tails, or going into labor on the subway, there is only one that I actually have power over. For psychological reasons, it is important to me to have permanent residence status in the United States before I give birth—not because, god forbid, I am making a lasting commitment, but because living on a four-year renewable visa is too temporary an arrangement even for me. Besides, without a green card, I can't borrow money. Toward the end of the year, my attorney prepares the last of the paperwork for submission to U.S. Citizenship and Immigration Services and tells me to make an appointment with a doctor.

All prospective green card holders have to be tested for diseases, an echo of Ellis Island–era protocols that requires me, one rainy day in early November, to haul my massive bulk resentfully downtown to the "green card doctor." I am so accustomed, by now, to my swanky hospital uptown that as I look around the clinic, I realize I am experiencing something that, should further evidence be needed, testifies to my assimilation into American society: health insurance snobbery.

Before the doctor comes in, the nurse asks me to remove the bottom half of my clothing and cover myself with a sheet.

"Why?" I ask.

"To check for STDs."

"You're kidding, right?"

The doctor enters.

"All righty!" he says, registers my face (thunderous) and my belly (gargantuan) and, turning to his nurse, says quickly, "OK, let's not do the STD test. It would be *unlikely*." Instead, he takes a perfunctory look in my eyes and mouth, signs the forms, tells me to get a bunch of shots, and lets me go, whereupon I dash up through Manhattan to Grand Central Terminal. Some people meet their lovers under the famous clock on the station concourse; I meet my immigration lawyer for a handover of green card paperwork before she takes the last Friday night fast train to Connecticut. "You look well," she says and peers a bit closer. She is older than me, the mother of three children and a successful attorney. "Are you frightened?"

I am taken aback by her directness. "Yes. Really frightened."

"It's normal. After the birth, you'll cry the first night and be out of your mind with fear. Then, the next morning, you'll feel like you rule the universe."

The station's heavy foot traffic flows around us and I am suddenly flooded with gratitude. It hasn't been a spouse I have missed in all this, I realize, but a mother—not my own mother specifically, because I can't imagine even being here if she was alive. But the idea of a mother, the person who doesn't wait to be asked; who sees past my bravado to the cowering wreck underneath and then tells me the universe is mine. "My other piece of advice," says my lawyer, "since everyone I know is having twins, is if you see something you like in Buy Buy Baby and there are only three left, buy two."

On my way home and in my apartment that evening, I feel my mind extend an invitation to itself to weep and feel bad. My mother isn't here and will never meet these babies. In her absence, I will have to rely on the paid help of strangers. I will be denied the joy her joy would have given me. I don't remember if I cried, which makes me think I didn't, but either way, it was the idea of my mother's absence that hurt, rather than the absence itself. I don't miss her more on rainy days or on Sunday afternoons and I don't miss her more now than before I was pregnant. It would be like saying I am more aware of my arm at some times than at others. I'm not. It's always there, being an arm, just as my mother's death is always there in the space behind my ribs, unobtrusive and immutable. If anything, there is a direct line from her life to the life of my babies that makes her seem closer, not further away. I think of her, I think of them, and it is impossible not to be happy.

SO FAR, most of my preparations for the birth haven't, I don't think, been that different from those of pregnant women with spouses. I go to baby store Web sites and panic at all the terrible junk I am expected to buy. ("Snack tray for a double stroller": essential or optional? "High-waisted postnatal support pants," ditto.) I try to prepare for the unpreparable. At my friend Sheila's fortieth birthday party in Brooklyn, I have a single glass of Prosecco and pose for a photo with Oliver, our arms slung round each other, grinning. My belly is poking out through the curtains of my leopard print coat, which, at seven months pregnant and under cover of absurdity, I finally have the confidence to wear. I stare at the photo for a long time on the subway ride home. The lighting is dark, so that apart from my belly, it could have been taken at any point over the last eighteen years. "You know you're in the frame for male role model?" I yelled at Oliver before leaving, above the roar of the bar.

"I'll be around so much," he roared back, "you'll have to ask me to leave."

One Saturday morning, a lovely man I find on the Internet comes to my apartment to put together the crib. In the made-for-TV movie of this pregnancy, I would be shot leaning sadly in the doorway of my office-turned-nursery, looking down at his builder's crack and wondering where my life had gone wrong. (L, who is very handy with a screwdriver, could've done the job, but neither of us had ever fully recovered from the Disastrous Joint Assembly of the Bed from West Elm. Better to get someone in.)

The question of a baby nurse is harder to fathom. This is less fraught a decision in New York than in London, where the very word "nanny" is used to beat up women who work, casting them as a bunch of spoiled Edwardians palming their kids off on the help—a characterization from which, naturally, fathers are entirely exempt. In New York, there are fewer class implications involved in hiring a nanny, but the race implications are stark; the vast majority of nannies in New York are black or Hispanic; the vast majority of employers are white. It's also weird, the idea of sharing a living space with someone I've only just met when my boobs will be out half the time. None of our parents had baby nurses; most of them didn't even have child care and this leap into Nannyland is as big and peculiar as any I've felt. It hasn't escaped my notice that, while living with L was apparently too much for me, for the first month of my children's lives I will be living with a sixty-year-old Caribbean lady instead.

Phyllis is from Grenada, recommended by a friend of L's, with twenty-seven years' experience of looking after newborn twins. I don't understand how someone can, for twenty-seven years, barely have an unbroken night's sleep and still be alive, but here she is on my sofa, her natty snow-leopard print beret cocked to one side, telling me about her infant charges, about her relationship with "Jesus Christ our Lord" and, with a little digging, about the ex-husband she banished to a flat in her basement before changing the locks on her doors. Phyllis's references, when I check them out, come from a variety of people: a hard-pressed legal aid lawyer in the Bronx; some very posh people in banking; and an Englishwoman on the Upper East Side who tells me how marvelous Phyllis was when they took her yachting off Bermuda, so that I worry she'll be slumming it in my modest two-bedroom. I also wonder if I can do without her.

My dad and Marion, his partner, will fly in as close to the birth as they can. L will be around mornings, evenings and weekends, although not overnight, with her own son to care for, and Oliver will look in several times a week. With one baby, this patchwork would probably suffice. But with two, particularly if I'm recovering from surgery, it strikes me as completely impossible. I'm freelance. I have no paid maternity leave and need to get back to work for at least a few hours a day within as short a time period as possible. There's no way around it; I'll have to bite the bullet.

I interview one other candidate, who doesn't have a cute beret or smile once during the course of our hour-long conversation and then I call Phyllis. I'm a little worried about the god thing, but I'm confident we can work around it. "I knew you were the one when you told me you locked your husband in the basement," I tell her.

"Well, that's not quite what I—" protests Phyllis. Then she clacks her tongue and roars with laughter.

THERE IS ONE very big difference between the preparations I am making and those being made by the other pregnant women in my pre-natal group, and that is the extent to which I have to budget for my own death. I have no siblings, no close cousins, and my dad is in his seventies. I am also in the wrong country. I once got very, very drunk with a BBC camera crew at a hotel in Beirut and the next day thought I was dying. When I called Merope in London to say good-bye, I came over all *English Patient* (if Kristin Scott Thomas had been dressed by North Face and made out with a BBC cameraman) and made her promise to repatriate my body. "Don't let them leave me in Lebanon," I said. "I want my ashes to be scattered in England."

"I think you're still drunk, my love."

"Promise me."

"I will. Now try to throw up and I'll call again in ten minutes."

Nothing much in my attitude on this subject has changed. England is home and will always be home and when I think about dying, not only do I want my ashes to be shipped back, I can't help wanting my babies to go with them. This is completely irrational, wholly impractical and highly offensive to L. Still, I can't help it. If I leave my two orphans in a place I still find so strange, how will they ever find their way home?

To defer having to make a decision, I take out a $1 million life insurance policy, surprisingly cheap when you squeak in under forty, and it even covers me for suicide—I burst out laughing when the sales agent tells me this on the phone. "Well, that certainly expands the range of my options," I say. She doesn't laugh.

"You'll be sixty-nine when this policy expires," she says and I abruptly stop cackling.

Then I call a good friend in London. "Who's your kids' guardian if you and Scott die?"

"Aaaaaargh! It's Scott's parents at the moment, but they're too old."

"But he has a sister, right?"

"Yeah, but I won't let her have them because her husband's a fucking selfish fuck. He wouldn't do right by my girls. Actually, I was thinking of asking you. But I guess your plate is full."

Everyone I call that week has the same story. Most of us had children so late our parents are too old to be made their guardians. Eventually, I talk to L.

"I'm not sure if leaving them in the United States is what I want," I say.

"What do you mean?"

I sense danger and try to walk back. "I mean, it's just that if they stay here, they'll have less of a sense of who I was than in England."

"Are you kidding me?"

The rest of the conversation doesn't go well. My contingency plan—to ask my friend Leila if she'll take them if I die during their first year, after which I'll revisit the decision—annoys L so wildly that for a while, whenever I asked her to do something, she says, "Why don't you ask Leila?" And of course she is right, not only because I am being childish and unreasonable, but because it is not my decision to make. My children will fall in love with the person they see all the time and long before they speak, the decision will speak for itself.

At Thanksgiving, L braces for impertinent questions about my pregnancy from conservative elements in her family. None comes. Everyone is lovely and tolerant and excited about the babies, and this is how it seems to go. Even those of my friends who, conceiving in circumstances similar to mine, suffered the initial dispproval of relatives, watched as they changed their minds once a baby was born. You have to be a spectacular cunt to set eyes on a child and reject it on the basis of provenance.

IN EARLY DECEMBER, L throws me a baby shower—"Why don't you get Leila to throw you one?"—at our local Chinese restaurant and I wear a crown and play dumb games and eat my own body weight in lo mein and, given how grudging I used to be about this kind of event, am touched by how many people turn up. The following week, I eat the last of the leftovers before the fetal nonstress test, and the babies are so high on MSG it takes three hours to get two adequate readings. (These tests, which monitor the babies' heart rates and are conducted weekly in the last months of my pregnancy, for some reason aren't routinely covered by my insurance and so one of the doctors arranges for the paperwork to be sent to his office and adjusted before being sent on.) After the test, I go downstairs to be looked over by Dr. Y. "Two good, brave babies," he says, beaming.

My final ultrasound of the year falls just after Christmas. I am six weeks from the due date and still have a lot to get done. The technician looks at the screen. "What do you have as the deepest vertical pocket on A?" she says to her colleague. He frowns, says something I don't catch and leaves the room. Someone else comes in. Everyone gathers by the monitor while I look at the ceiling and try to figure out whether to have lunch on the East Side, or save myself ten dollars and eat out of the fridge when I get home.

Finally, a fourth doctor comes in and tells me to get dressed. "Could you follow me, please?" he says. I feel a spike of alarm. We walk to his office, where Dr. Y is waiting.

"They have to come out," says Dr. Y.

"Oh my god."

The placenta for the smallest baby is working only intermittently; if it stops altogether she'll die. "This is not an emergency," says Dr. Y calmly, "but it is . . . fairly urgent." He tells me he has time in his calendar the following day, New Year's Eve, or the day after that. Even in my panic, I realize that New Year's Day is the very worst day of the year to have surgery. In any case, I don't want to make Baby A wait.

"Let's do it tomorrow," I say, trembling.

"Three p.m.?"

"OK."

"We'll see you then."

How can he be so casual? Why isn't anyone screaming or calling the newspapers? As I stagger out of the room, one of the doctors smiles and jokes that I should look on the bright side. Having them before the New Year will bring significant tax breaks. "Call your accountant!" he says.

THIRTEEN

Neonatal

I LIE ON MY BED looking up at the ceiling. I've changed my mind, I think vaguely. I've thoroughly enjoyed this pregnancy; it's been interesting and challenging and wonderful in every way, but I've had enough now and would like to go home. In fact, this entire twenty-year experiment in adult living has been more than sufficient and it's high time my parents came to collect me. I picture myself as a child, walking down my old street on a summer afternoon, holding my mum's hand as the sunlight dips in and out of the trees above our heads. In some obscure way I know we are sailing toward death in this scene, but it always reassures me; the grip of her hand, the flicker of the sun, the sense that whatever else happens, some part of me is fortified against the unknown, inside this moment forever.

At thirty-four weeks' gestation, the babies are only three weeks shy of full term for twins, but because of the problem with the placenta, the doctors believe the smaller of the two babies might have stopped developing at thirty-two weeks. The surgery tomorrow is not a marginal call. It is a vital measure to preserve the life of the baby, and after the initial panic, the main thing I feel is relief: not that the doctors caught the problem in time, or that their prognosis is optimistc. I'm relieved that the threat to the baby is so unequivocal my insurers can't possibly challenge it.

It crosses my mind that I will never know what it's like to give birth. I'm not sorry to miss out on the pain, but a small part of me regrets missing out on the symbolism. Surely the only appropriate way to honor a transition of this size is by crawling down the labyrinth of labor? Without it, I fear, I'll get whiplash. I look at the two empty bassinets at the end of my bed and my mind flips. How can a person go from having no children to having two children in the space of twenty minutes and with no discernible effort on her part? "I only hope they're not bald," I say on the phone to Oliver, trying to jolly myself back to normality. "No offense."

"Thanks a lot."

Oliver is at his parents' home in the north of England. Merope is in Cornwall, in the west. My dad is in London and cancels his plans for New Year's to stay in and sit by the phone. He offers to come straight to New York, but I don't want him in the air while I'm having surgery; I can't add fear of his plane going down to everything else. At L's that night, after she asks what I want for my last supper and we order a curry, I tell her to ask her mother to come across town the following day to watch her son for as long as proves necessary.

"I'm so happy you'll be there," I say.

"It's only because everyone else is in England."

"No, it isn't. I would want you to be there whatever."

As I say this, I realize it's true. The hospital permits only one adult to be with the mother in the operating theater, and if my own mother were alive, I wonder if I would push L out into the corridor. My mother would be champing at the bit to be involved, but she had an innate sense of fairness and I think she would have seen this as wrong. It feels wrong to me, too. I went through the inseminations without L and didn't care for her company during the scans. I gritted my teeth and got through the amnio alone, because I found it easier to do it this way. Fear pushes me inward, joy pushes me out, and while I am as frightened of having these babies as of anything, it's a different kind of fear; not a shrinking but an opening out. I have been so stringent in ensuring I can do this alone, perhaps the reward is I don't always have to.

At some point during dinner, I raise my eyes from my plate to find L looking at me, eyes wide.

"I know," I say. It's a law of relationship physics that you can't both feel the same thing at the same time, and in the face of her fear, I feel myself strengthen.

"Do you want to stay up here, tonight?" she says.

"No, I'll go home in a minute. This is my last ever night alone in my apartment."

Downstairs, I pack all the things they tell you to take to the hospital and for which no one has any use when they arrive: dressing gown, "boiled sweets," industrial-size underpants, "photos of your loved ones," as if I were emigrating, not going to a place twenty minutes from my house, to which three hundred restaurants and two branches of Duane Reade deliver. Then I call Phyllis, the baby nurse, to tell her the girls are coming early and she should stand by. "Praise the Lord!" she says. "He has a plan for us all."

The next morning is crisp and bright, a perfect December day. On the corner of the street, L hails a taxi. "Isn't this great?" she says.

"What?"

"Not being in a rush. God, I love C-sections."

When we reach the far side of the park, we hit traffic and she turns to me.

"Can I say it?"

"I feel bad for the guy."

"Come on."

"But it's a scheduled C-section!"

"Go on, let me."

I sigh. "OK."

L leans forward in her seat and bangs on the driver's window. "Hey!" she yells. "HEY! Excuse me? Sir? Excuse me? Can you put your foot on the gas? She's having a baby!"

FOR THE NEXT few hours everything feels like a dream. The balloons in the waiting area, bobbing over the large family groups patiently waiting for news. The rock star doctor walking past and coming over to see me. "How many weeks?" he says.

"Thirty-four."

He nods and gives me a hug. "It's time."

It is a good day to give birth. The hospital has a giddy, public holiday atmosphere to it that feels like a celebration put on just for me. Dr. Y comes out in his scrubs to say hi. Anticipation makes L and me giggly. She buys a salad and eats it ostentatiously in front of me, which is hilarious because I can't eat or drink. When we enter the delivery ward and approach the front desk, we nearly trip over a woman on her hands and knees, crawling around on the floor and moaning with labor pains while nurses race down the corridor to reach her. "Aren't you glad you're having a C-section?" whispers L and we have to break into a run not to be heard laughing.

In the prep room, the nurse putting the line into my hand keeps missing the vein and having to redo it. "I can't get anything right today!" she says, giggling, an amazing admission of liability in these parts, and which in our own giddy mood strikes us as mad and delightful. The nurses hand L some scrubs and she puts them on and for the next twenty minutes we take photos of ourselves with a selfie stick and behave as if we were on a school trip to a maternity ward, blissfully unimplicated by any of it. In the next cubicle, we hear a couple—a "regular couple," as I know we both think of it—murmuring to each other in low, anxious tones. It must be astounding and beautiful to give birth to a baby with the look-what-we-made aspect of having the dad by one's side. But there is something beautiful and astounding about this, too. It isn't, surely, supposed to be this fun.

Eventually, the ditzy nurse comes back in and says the surgical team is ready for me. L and I sober up. She squeezes my hand. "See you in a minute."

I am generally an insufficiently grateful person. I am grateful for health, and love, and various accidents of birth, but I know I underplay luck to flatter my own industry. Now, perched on the edge of the operating table as the anesthetist prepares the spinal block, I feel a deep, overwhelming sense of gratitude. I have told myself these babies are mine because they were meant to be mine, but behind this conviction I feel the shadow of how things might have turned out. Now that they're here, the enormity of their presence can be measured, in part, by the enormity of imagining their absence.

"This is the worst bit," says the doctor and for a second I shake so violently he has to wait for me to stop.

"It's so cold in here!"

"It is," he says kindly. Then he swabs my back and there is a deep, sharp pain. I lie down and L comes in, followed by Dr. Y and a handful of student doctors. Then three nurses from the neonatal intensive care unit wheel in the two incubators.

It turns out the pain of the injection is not the worst thing. The worst thing is managing the fear—not that there will be anything wrong with the babies, but that the anesthetic won't work and I'll feel every cut.

"Can you feel this?" says the anesthetist, tapping me somewhere on the abdomen. I hesitate. What does it really mean to "feel"? I am aware he has tapped me; the vibration registers. But is that the same thing as "feeling"? Might one be said to have an awareness of something that falls below an articulable level, but that still reaches the threshold of feeling? Luckily, I am a writer and can describe subtle states. "Kind of," I say. "Not really."

"On a scale of one to ten, how acutely can you feel this?" he says and I say a number at random—"Six?"—then he moves up and does it again. We carry on this way for several moments, the doctor tapping my flesh while I throw out numbers at random, until he stops and says, "Good." I brace myself for the cut of the knife.

When I was delivered by C-section in 1975, my mother was knocked out with a general anesthetic and my dad wasn't allowed in the room. Now L is sitting on a stool by my head and the only propriety is a low screen drawn across my chest, so that neither of us can witness the carnage. There are strict rules about filming in the OR, presumably for legal reasons, but as Dr. Y leans in to start work, L pops out of her seat and begins taking photos over the screen with her phone. Abruptly, she sits down.

"How is it?"

"It's crazy."

I am suddenly euphoric. "I don't feel a thing!"

A moment later, there is a tremendous pressure, as if I were being pulled apart lengthways by two teams of horses. L stands up to take more photos and Dr. Y's voice carries across the OR like a school principal spotting disorder in the back row. "Sit down!" he booms. She sits down.

This will sound absurd, but right up until the last moment a small part of me thinks, what if all this is a mistake? What if it's a phantom pregnancy? What if Dr. Y turns to me and says, surprise! There's nothing in there, of course you're not pregnant! Did you really think you could have a baby without the machinery of marriage, or long-term commitment, or compromise with someone else's parenting ideas, or an identifiable father, for god's sake? Did you think that, by turning up at a clinic, signing a few forms and handing over your credit card, you could dodge millennia of evolution, not to mention custom, convention and common decency? Go home, buy yourself a cat and never speak of this again.

At 4:17 p.m., a tiny, fierce cry fills the room. Baby A, whose existence I doubted even while I feared for her life, is removed from the basement of my body. I burst into tears. L grips my hand. A moment later, Baby B comes out and L leaps from her seat in the direction of the babies while Dr. Y, turning to his students, holds a quick pop quiz over my guts. Then the nurses bring over the babies to show me.

L gets all of this illegally on camera. It's not footage I can watch too often. The babies, two flat-faced Gloworms covered in gel, are blotchy and impossibly alive. I am insane on the gurney, head turned to one side, grinning drunkenly at my two girls. Over and over I say it, in the manner of a woman shortly to be given more drugs: "Oh my god, I can't believe they're both blond."

A FEW MINUTES LATER, one of the nurses says gently, "We need to take them downstairs." Both babies are breathing on their own, but they are very small and will need constant monitoring. I lie in the recovery room and, after begging L to go to the drinks machine in the corridor, throw back the best can of Coke of my life. A few hours later, I'm wheeled up to a room on the maternity ward and L goes downstairs to the NICU. She comes back with phone footage more miraculous than the moon landing. Baby B is in an open bassinet with monitors on her chest. Baby A, the smaller of the two, is in her tank hooked up to a nest of wires. "Hey, Baby A!" says L softly in the background, while the baby looks around as if she's just been pushed from an airplane at thirty-five thousand feet. "Oh, no, wait—you're Baby B! Hey, Baby B! How are you doing?"

I used to see pictures of premature babies in the newspapers and wonder how their parents could love them. I don't mean because preterm infants are ugly. It's just that when they're that tiny they don't seem to be human in scale. It would, I used to think, be like trying to make an adequate pet of an insect. I assumed that in place of love, the mothers must be relying on pity and hormones. Well, ha. Within moments of the birth I feel a tide move within me. The entire universe whittles down to a bright knot in my core. I think of Merope after the birth of her first baby all those years ago, saying, "It's like being punched in the face by love." I think of those stories of women who overturn burning cars to get their children out. I have seen the babies for only a few moments and I am desperate, livid, raging with love.

L sits by my side, late into that night and for hours over the coming days. She brings me pizza, and chicken soup, and fried chicken from the deli. She instructs me on how to go "off-menu" and get better food out of the hospital kitchen. She brings in her son who is not my son but who is drawn closer to me by the birth of my children. I have yet to do a single ounce of parenting, but something discreet between L and me shifts. A balance is achieved, not only between the two of us, but back through the generations. "You know," she says, returning to me after visiting the babies downstairs, "their hair isn't blond. It's red."

The morning after the birth, I get in a wheelchair and ask to be pushed down to the locked ward of the NICU. I am barefoot, in my hospital gown, shuffling over to the incubators in the company of half a dozen other women, all crazy on drugs and anxiety. On the way back up, the orderly accidentally wheels me into a garbage can and an hour later, after taking more painkillers, I put on sneakers and, leaning at a forty-five-degree angle to protect my incision, walk down to the NICU myself.

They are not the tiniest babies on the unit, but they are still not much bigger than the palm of my hand. How long they stay in the hospital will depend on how well they gain weight and whether any developmental problems come to light. Over the coming days, the bigger of the two's heart rate will occasionally dip below safety thresholds and set off a piercing alarm, adding a mandatory five days to her stay. The smaller of the two will have a feeding tube inserted into her nose and contract jaundice, so that for hours of the day she will lie under a photo-therapy lamp wearing cumbersome goggles. She hates the goggles and cries pitifully, pushing at them uselessly with arms no wider than my thumbs, while I stand stricken by the side of her tank. A nurse helps me to remove her, holding her wires like a bridal train so they don't catch on the chair, and there she lies in my arms like a featherless bird, the veins on her eyelids picked out in blue.

Four days after the birth, I walk out of the hospital alone, carrying only what I brought in with me, plus the Chanel gift bag the maternity ward issues to every new mother, while that particular sponsorship deal holds. In the taxi, clutching my middle as we go over bumps, I test out a weird new sensation. I am here, but I am also elsewhere. I am in this taxi alone but a part of me remains at the hospital. For what feels like the first time in years, I'm not conflicted about what matters most. Everything that mattered a week ago still matters, but this new thing matters more.

That evening, I will go back to the NICU to see the babies for three hours, but until then I'm not sure what to do. At home, I skirt the doorman to avoid having to give an account of myself, then hover in the vestibule of my apartment. Because the babies came early I still have work on my desk and, reaching for the old masochistic buzz, shuffle down the hallway to my office. On the way, I glance into my bedroom and catch sight of the two empty cribs at the foot of my bed. I put my hands on my knees and sob.

IT IS A STRANGE INTRODUCTION to motherhood. For the next two weeks, I get eight hours' sleep a night, more than I've had for months. In the mornings, I go up to L's apartment before she heads off to work, then come downstairs to deal with insurance and admin. The more forms I can fill out, the more substantial the babies' existence will be and the stronger purchase they will have on this world. This is how it feels. I gather together what they need for their American passports and look into what they'll need for the British ones. I even register their births with the British Foreign Office, an entirely unnecessary measure that requires an amazing amount of subsidiary evidence, including my dad's birth certificate and my parents' marriage certificate, and all of which keeps me going for days. Every day I ring my dad with an update on the babies and tell him to hold on for more news before flying. There is nothing anyone can do but wait.

In the afternoons, I get a taxi across town to the NICU. The nurses jokingly call it the most expensive babysitting service in the world, and for all the anxiety on the ward, it is a comforting place. Monitors beep and winter light fills the room, filtering in across the East River. The nurses are cheerful. "Hey, Red," they say to Jane, Baby A, whose hair is now a deep auburn. "Hey, Dee Dee," they say to Baby B. "She's so smiley!" They handle these tiny creatures with deftness and love and handle the parents with the same loving certainty. One day, one of the doctors tries to put a central line into a minuscule vein in Jane's arm while she lets out a high, bleating scream and I pace in the background, trying not to put my head through a wall. "Do you need to take a walk?" says the nurse, looking up at me sharply, and I go out to the waiting area to stare at the fish tanks. At nine p.m., I go home for another decent night's sleep.

Toddlers are too germy to be allowed in the unit, so L gets a babysitter and comes to sit with us in the evenings. Sympathy among the families around each incubator is absolute. There are some disheveled Brits on my ward, who look as if they were surprised by an early arrival on holiday, and whose insurance coverage I worry about. There are a lot of large, multigenerational religious families, both Muslim and Orthodox

Jewish, all of whom deal unflinchingly with the number of naked boobs on display. (We are supposed to call a nurse to put screens up when we breast-fed, but most of us are too distracted to bother. Jane is still too small for the breast, but Dee Dee is big enough, although I manage to breast-feed her only one time in three. Trying to breast-feed a premature baby is like trying to get a kitten to blow up a beach ball.)

Success is measured in tiny increments of weight gain and the size and contents of their diapers. When one of my babies does a poo that weighs more than some babies on the unit I feel like I've won the Olympics. One day, I am feeding Dee Dee when an alarm call goes off at a neighboring incubator. Within seconds, a team of doctors have crossed the ward to reach him and yank closed the curtains. That evening the mother emerges looking dreadful. "I don't know if you . . . Did you see what happened this afternoon?" she says to me.

"Yes," I say. "It sounded awful." Her baby, who was born at twenty-four weeks and has a host of life-threatening complications, had gone into cardiac arrest, but they had managed to revive him. "A bad day," she says. She looks at Dee Dee in my arms and smiles faintly. "I just hope they don't remember any of this."

Mostly, we don't talk about the bad stuff. "Lovely name," says one mother to another. Or, "So much hair!" Or, "She looks bigger today!" There are social lunches in the meeting room, and classes on how to care for your preemie, and a breast pump room where, after pumping, we mark the bags of milk with our babies' names and put them in a fridge in the ward. When someone brings in a car seat to take her baby home, everyone cheers, but the truth is we all have mixed feelings about leaving. I am simultaneously desperate to get my babies home and terrified of being alone with them, without the safety net of monitors and a room full of doctors down the hall. How will I know if something is wrong if there isn't an alarm to inform me?

One afternoon, a nurse brings in a violin and goes ward to ward, playing tunes for the babies. She does "Swing Low, Sweet Chariot" and Pachelbel's Canon, and Dvořák's New World Symphony, and "Danny Boy." Here and there she hits a bum note, which I tell myself off for noticing. At the end of the set, she has her revenge. The last tune in her repertoire is "Over the Rainbow," and as she draws to a wobbly conclusion, every woman in the room bows her head over her tiny, wire-covered baby and gently, comprehensively loses it.

When I get in the next day, the nurse tells me someone rang the ward that morning asking after my babies. "He said it was 'Dad,'" she says.

"What?"

"Yeah. I didn't think that was right. I went generic on him and said the babies were beautiful and got off the line."

"British or American?"

"American. Could it have been your father?"

"No, he wouldn't call here. And anyway he's British."

I have a sensation of jump jets firing up in my brain. Whoever he is, I will find him and eliminate him, even if that means paying the ultimate price. (Not jail, obviously, but being depicted by Shannen Doherty in a made-for-TV movie called something like *A Mother's Revenge*.)

"It was probably a mistake," says the nurse. "Men occasionally ring in not knowing the names of their own babies. And we have a lot of twins."

"Well, whoever he was I'm glad he's not my husband. He sounds shit."

It never does get resolved. I let it go, along with every other concern outside the growth of the babies. They are fed on a three-hour schedule, and as they grow stronger, so I grow more presentable. One day, I even turn up at the hospital in clothes I haven't slept in. Development is measured in hours and days, so that when a new dad comes sprinting through the double doors, chasing an incubator, wild with terror and what I imagine to be his wife's words ringing in his ears—"Follow that baby!"—it seems to me to be a scene from a previous life. When I pass women in the corridor just down from the labor ward—sockless, shoeless, blasted, insane—I look at them with the fondness of someone recalling ancient history.

There had been a moment, on the second night after the babies were born, when I had sat in my hospital bed looking out of the window. Across the East River was Roosevelt Island and beyond that the power station in Long Island City. It is an arresting view; the river, the expanse of sky, the cooling towers in the distance. L had come and gone for the evening. I'd had my dinner and would be alone until a nurse came in at three a.m. to give me more pain meds. The night before, I had felt my mood crash in just the way my lawyer had warned me, a dread so vast— what had I done? How would I manage?—I could only turn my face to the wall and hope it would pass. The next night it was gone and I sat looking across the water, the sky darkening while somewhere two floors beneath me, doctors looked after my babies. After two weeks in the NICU, the babies would be discharged with a clean bill of health and L would come to drive us all home. Phyllis would move in, and a month later, move out. I would cry from lack of sleep and frustration. On nights like this, I would lie looking out at the apartment block opposite, wondering if dawn would ever come and if the babies, both still under five pounds, would ever get any bigger or sleep for more than three hours at a stretch. During the day, I would watch TV while they slept, and cry at the slightest hint of cruelty or violence on-screen. I would produce too little milk, then too much. My dad would fly in and hold the babies for the first time and the joy of his joy would be one of the great moments of life. L's son would come down every day to kiss the babies, and on the weekend, the three of us would spend two nights upstairs. Oliver would come, Dan would come, and Phyllis would come back three days a week, but there would never be enough hands. I would love the feeling of being in a bubble with my babies and occasionally fear I'd go mad from it.

People would go overboard remarking on how much the girls looked like me, something I enjoyed but also sensed was an awkward effort to obscure the fact of the donor. In fact, one did look like me and one looked to a startling extent like my mother, with the same hair and eyes and planes of her face, although they both have dimples and long lashes, neither of which comes from my side. More than anything, they look like themselves.

There would be moments of the purest, whitest terror; when one seemed to be choking on her spit-up and the other slipped from my hand in the tub. I would blame L for not coming downstairs enough and blame Phyllis for coming in late. Then I would go upstairs and long to be home alone with my babies and breathe a sigh of relief when Phyllis left for the week. I would watch in utter shock as my children fell in love with L and my love for her son tangled up with my love for my babies and lost the last of its tentative air. There was no word, still, for what we were to each other, but it felt solid, and implacable, and real.

Across the river, the lights in the apartments of Roosevelt Island went on and I felt a baseline within myself rising. There would be hard days and harder nights. There would be a million decisions to make, large and small. But that night, looking out from my hospital bed, I felt only the certainty of the room and my stillness within it, the future pressing in with a force I returned. At six a.m. the next morning I went downstairs to see the babies. I was still shuffling at a forty-five-degree angle, my smock open at the back, huge hospital pants poking out and gray hospital socks pulled up from my sneakers. As I walked in, the nurse looked up and smiled.

"Hey, Mamma," she said.

Epilogue

ONE BABY IS SLIPPING through the leg of the high chair. The other has flopped forward in her seat and is gumming the dirty edge of the table. The café is full but we're in a quiet corner, where I hope the waiter won't notice the mess.

"Do you need help?" says a woman, passing us on her way out, with a look I have grown accustomed to over the last six months—part admiration, part you poor cow.

"No, I have it, but thanks." With one hand, I grab the baby who's slipping and yank her back into place, while jamming the other hand between her sister's gums and the table. Thus balanced, I lean forward and take a slurp of my latte.

It is midmorning in late spring on a day I don't have help with the babies and I am happy to be out of the house. For the first four months, I barely left my apartment. I watched a lot of TV. I napped when the girls napped and pumped so much breast milk the freezer is jammed with it, yellowing in hard plastic sleeves like the flavor of Popsicle nobody wants. I forced myself to acclimatize to getting by on our own. The Sunday the babies came home from the hospital, I called Phyllis and told her not to come in until Monday. "Are you sure?" she said anxiously. "I can come over now."

"No, I need to do a night on my own or I'll never want you to leave." That evening, after spending the afternoon caring for the babies with L and her son, I sent them home, too. "Call me in the night if you need to," she said.

"OK."

"You sure you don't want to come upstairs with us?"

"No. We'll be fine."

"OK." She pulled a face of comic alarm, as if seeing me off at the edge of a desert. "Bye."

"Bye."

I returned to sit on the sofa, where the babies lay in their rockers before me. Cradled in receptacles made for babies up to four times their size, they looked like the victims of a bizarre science fiction experiment, in which human beings had been shrunk to the size of large earrings. Their onesies gaped at the arms. Their hats slipped over their eyes. While one baby slept, the other looked steadily up at me before flicking her eyes to take in the room. Then her gaze returned to meet mine. "Hello," I said.

Women, particularly married women who have just had a baby, ask me incredulously about the math of one parent versus two newborns. I have no answer. I did it, and afterward I forgot how I did it. Terror made me nimble. I ate a lot of Milky Ways. After that first night, when

I picked up the rockers one by one and carried them through to my bedroom, putting one by the side of my bed and one at the foot, I had Phyllis for the month, and after she left, although things were terrible at night, they were terrible within the realm of the manageable. That first night alone was the only time, with the exception of the mood plunge I had forty-eight hours after their birth, when I thought, this is too hard, I can't do it. It was dark in the room save for the purple glow of the night light and I couldn't get a grip on my fear. Every time I thought I had it under control, a new wave rose up to engulf me. At some point, after a stretch of high bleating cries that nothing I did would assuage, I got up to unlock my front door; clearly none of us would survive the night, and in the morning, the police would need to get in to recover our bodies. This habit continued long after Phyllis had left; I would take my chances with the burglars for the sake of not being locked in with my fears. Anyway, the real killers were here with me already.

They were so small for so long. No matter how hot my apartment, their skin always looked so mottled and cold. Even with Phyllis there, the onslaught of pump-feed-change-repeat was brutal, although her presence made that first month the easiest it would be for a long time. There is a comic novel to be written called *My Month with Phyllis,* in which a thirty-nine-year-old white woman and a sixtysomething Caribbean woman become unlikely flatmates and friends. It shouldn't have worked but it did. She was kind, and funny, and eccentric in ways I found charming. We overlooked each other's foibles. Phyllis overlooked the fact that I didn't shower more than one day in four and that whatever I was doing with the lady upstairs probably went against the teachings of Christ, and I overlooked the fact that Satan visited her in dreams and that she gave all her wages to a diet doctor in Coney Island. I tried not to be bitter about this, but it was hard. Slowly, in weekly cash increments of twenty-five hundred dollars, I was buying Dr. Botkin a summer home.

"What are you doing, Phyllis?" I asked grumpily one night, catching sight of her on the sofa, head bowed, fiddling with something behind her ears. The babies were side by side on her lap, dozing after a feed.

"I'm doing my ball bearings," she said and explained Dr. Botkin's method of implanting tiny silver balls behind his patient's ears, which they were instructed to rotate every night to achieve weight loss. When that didn't work, she went on a cabbage diet, infusing the apartment with the smell of a hospital kitchen. "Really? Phyllis? Cabbage?" When Satan visited her, she cried out, "Devil, be gone!" and he left. Sometimes I got up in the night and we'd sit side by side on the sofa, each feeding a baby, and sometimes I slept through, going into her room at five a.m. to collect the girls for their first feed of the day.

"Another rough night?" I asked when Phyllis emerged several hours later, startling in the hallway in her Victorian nightgown. "How's Satan?"

She clicked her tongue. "You." When I came downstairs from L's one evening, upset after a disagreement, she gave me a hug and said kindly, "Relationships are hard."

As I recall, the disagreement with L had been about Phyllis. If L and I thought we'd come up with a clever way to downsize human need, we were wrong. I should have known this from the jealousies I felt after the birth of her son, when I resented everyone else L looked to for help. Just because we weren't doing this together didn't mean third parties were welcome.

"Can't you tell her to take five in her room when I come down?" said L.

"I need her. I don't want to be rude."

"Why don't you just ask?"

This was the ghost of an old argument, as much about L's directness versus my circuitous Englishness as it was about accommodating each other's needs. In those first weeks and months, it was one of the few arguments we had. There were no fights about who should get up in the night because, once Phyllis left, that person would always be me. No one's career stalled at the expense of the other's and there was no bickering about who paid for what. And yet while "no one to resent" could be the unofficial motto of the single mother by choice, it isn't really true. In my experience, there is always someone to resent—the stress and exhaustion has to come out somewhere—and if I wasn't resenting L for leaving when I wanted her to stay, I was resenting Phyllis for taking too long when she went downstairs to do laundry, and L was resenting me for leaning on Phyllis. She had her own two-year-old; she was exhausted, too.

At the same time, I was aware that everything L did in those weeks was a gift, not a duty and I mostly received it as such. She ran around town picking up new bouncers and equipment that might help the gassier of the two babies sleep. She ordered boxes of preemie clothes that would actually fit and forced me to persevere with the smaller baby when she struggled to breast-feed. When I went upstairs to see her for twenty minutes in the evening, leaving the babies with Phyllis, we watched TV and played with her son, then she came downstairs to kiss the babies good night. She tickled Dee Dee's feet and nuzzled Jane's red hair. "She looks like me," said L teasingly.

"She does."

There are two versions of what happened in the weeks after Phyllis left and before the babies were stable enough to sleep through the night. One is an idyllic run of lazy afternoons, with snow at the window and a historical drama on TV, all three of us dozing to the whir of the breast pump. This was the bubble into which I was sometimes reluctant to admit L and that had occasionally made me happy when Phyllis took her days off. And there is another version of that time, which I have largely expunged from my memory. At four weeks old, the babies were still smaller than most newborns. Between seven and nine p.m. nightly but sometimes extending on toward midnight, one or the other of them screamed without pause. L would drop by to help, but had to excuse herself after an hour to put her own son to bed, after which it was like a scene from a horror movie. I would rock one baby in my arms until she settled, then put her down to pick up the other one, whereupon the one I'd put down started screaming again. This cycle rebooted over and over, until I lost all reason, putting down one baby and picking up another in such rapid succession that neither was soothed for a minute. I had a vision of myself rotating the babies like juggling balls, becoming madder and madder with each manic rotation. Occasionally, I got away with putting one baby in her bouncer and rocking it with my foot while sitting on the sofa with the other one. And sometimes I could wear one in a carrier on my front and cradle the other between my side and my forearm—the single advantage of their being so small—then walk around the room, jiggling them both. But neither of them liked these solutions, either being abandoned to the rocker or sharing my body space with her twin, and it tended only to prolong the agony. It was brutal and the worst thing about it was that it was brutal in what felt like a singular way. Just before the girls were born, I had joined a Facebook group made up of first-time twin moms in my area and, while Phyllis was still in residence, had been to the group's inaugural monthly dinner, where we all had two sips of wine and were instantly wasted. I avoided the group after that. The other women were lovely and it wasn't that I was ashamed of being a single parent, but they were all married, and once Phyllis left, my experiences felt so vastly different, they might as well have been twelve single men.

I should probably have persevered. It might have been helpful to talk, even if our experiences diverged. As it was, within weeks of the birth, I started to feel I couldn't justify dropping a hundred dollars on dinner once a month. I couldn't believe I had worried so much about the cost of conceiving the babies—which had come to less than the cost of getting my green card in the end—and barely given a thought to the costs once they were born.

"Yeah, but it's finite," said Merope. "You'll have no money for five years, and then they'll start school."

This might have been true in England. And while it was almost certainly true that, because of competition in the fertility market, the cost of getting pregnant had been cheaper in New York than it would have been in London, once the children were born, the American system felt staggeringly, punitively expensive. The monthly cost of health insurance for the three of us is half the cost of my mortgage again and won't expire when the children turn five. Unlike in the UK, there is no universal free dental care for kids. There is no universal free anything. It is grindingly hard to raise two kids on a single income in New York, and I say that as someone who is relatively prosperous.

After the first month, I couldn't afford Phyllis for twenty-four hours a day, but neither could I afford not to sleep or work, and so, until the babies got bigger, she agreed to come back for two nights and three days a week. That left me with five nights to manage alone and I moved out to the sofa during that time, the girls sleeping alongside me in their day cribs. I found this arrangement less isolating than being alone in the bedroom, and when they woke at one a.m., and two a.m., and three a.m., and four, I could kid myself that it was a less alarming time of night. No one ever died of fright at eight p.m. Only the darkness of the apartments across the street betrayed this lie and I would fixate on the odd light in a window—a shift worker, an insomniac, someone with a newborn, like me—and beam out signals of empathy and distress.

On Saturdays, I would take the rockers upstairs and spend the night on L's sofa, while she slept in her room with her son. By agreement, she didn't come out when they cried, unless the crying went on longer than the space of a feed. One Saturday, after a particularly bad run of sleepless nights when the longest either baby had slept was forty minutes, L came out at three a.m. looking alarmed. I was burping one of the babies so hard, she could hear the sound of the slaps through the wall.

"Give her to me," she said gently.

Describing all this makes it sound pretty appalling. But if it was shockingly hard, it was also shockingly simple. The babies' comfort was my comfort and I had no choice but to do it. When people say their kids give life meaning, what they mean, I think, is that this absence of choice, coupled with a love so huge it throws everything that came before into shade, can feel even on hard days—especially on hard days—a lot like destiny.

On the days Phyllis wasn't there, Oliver looked in, bringing lunch, and other friends with freelance schedules came, too. My dad and Marion came for three weeks. "I'm here to see my American grandchildren," said my dad proudly, when the immigration officer at JFK asked him for the purpose of his visit.

"They're not American," I said to L, later.

"Get over it," she said, "they're American."

Slowly, I figured out how to do things alone: how to shower (drag both bouncy seats into the bathroom with me, or leave the babies in the living room and wash for two minutes to the sound of their screaming); take them on the subway (wear one in the carrier and push the other in the single stroller); feed them simultaneously (sit on the floor between rockers, with a bottle of breast milk in each hand); and do everything I used to do with two hands—load the dishwasher, clean the bath, make an omelet—with one, because I always had a baby clamped to my hip. (I'm kidding about the bath, obviously. I never cleaned it.) When they both clamored for care, I picked them up under the armpits, one in each hand, so that by the time they were one, I was able to bench-press two toddlers with relative ease. Above all, in those winter months, I figured out how not to leave the house. In the early days, I truly believe the key to being a single mother of twins is to have everything delivered to your door.

There were a few things I couldn't work out. I worried endlessly about what to do in the event of a fire. Could I carry the two of them safely down seventeen flights of stairs on my own? Would I have time to put on the carrier, or is that the kind of thing that costs a woman and her babies their lives? Then, incredibly, there was a fire, smoke billowing in through the cracks of the elevator one morning as I traveled down with the babies to the lobby. When the doors opened, black smoke poured in and both babies began screaming and retching. I made a split-second decision: to go back up a burning building rather than expose their tiny lungs to one more mouthful of smoke, and as the elevator climbed, I called 911. Within minutes, half a dozen fire trucks were parked round the block. "You're OK, you're OK," said the operator, over and over, until a fireman banged on our door and said it was a blaze in the laundry room and they had put it out.

I was radioactive with tiredness, but in those early days I wasn't particularly lonely. This had as much to do with the babies as with L and my friends. Before they could talk and assert themselves as separate human beings, it sometimes felt as if the three of us functioned as one. When I had stomach flu one night and puked roughly every twenty minutes for eight hours, both babies were eerily silent. They understood.

Harder, much harder, was the period when they got older and combined the needs of babies with the complicated emotional needs of toddlers. At six months, we said an emotional good-bye to Phyllis and welcomed Jeanette, who'd care for them during the week so I could finally get back to working full time, and it was then, during the long evenings and weekends, that I was so lonely. Some days I wanted to run out into the street, throw myself at the first maternal-looking woman in late middle age, and demand she take me home and look after me. The girls were early talkers, and before they turned one, we entered the period of strict toddler religious law: "mummy hair" (down), "mummy shoes" (off), "mummy sit" (there). Spoons had to be the right color and placed on the right side of the plate. Different pacifiers were required for different times of day and night. There was a whole subsection concerning lids; if I forgot myself and ripped the lid off a yogurt rather than tearing it halfway, so the dictator-toddler could rip off the other half, that yogurt was rejected or hurled to the floor. On the other hand, if I didn't twist on the lid of the sippy cup with sufficient force, that cup was poison to their lips. Sometimes I was good-natured about this and sometimes I lost it, and I think I lost it more because there was no one else there.

L cut my girls' nails. I played endless games of cars with her son. As the girls got older, she taught them how to eat pizza like a New Yorker (hold it in one hand and curl it up at the edges), rather than a British person (fold it over or tear off individual bits, which makes L actively angry), and to drink seltzer with as much enthusiasm as milk. We were both reluctant to babysit for each other—after a long day, refereeing two toddlers and a three-year-old feels like the enactment of a medieval curse—which meant going out was expensive and hard. But we would sometimes swap kids for an afternoon for a change. And while we weren't parents to each other's children—the relationship was less intense than that, less inclined toward overprotection and free of the encumbrances of being the last word—as a result, we were often more fun and less cranky with each other's kids than with our own. My girls are part of me in a way that makes it very hard for me to imagine an alternative life in which they hadn't come to exist, but L's son is something else—an unexpected gift, a rare joy, a love I couldn't have foreseen.

He calls the girls "my babies," and sometimes, "my best friends." The girls call L by her name, as her son calls me by mine, and then something interesting happened. From the time she first spoke, my daughter Jane called me "Mummy-ya," and out of the blue one day when she was eighteen months old, she affixed the suffix "ya" to the end of L's name. It doesn't require a Ph.D. in linguistics to understand what she had done here. In the absence of a word for who L is in her life, she has intuited a family connection and come up with one. A year later, it's a linguistic rule she reserves for the three things she loves most in life: mummy(ya), L(ya) and the iPhone(ya).

To my amazement, my children are richer in people than I had been as a child. My dad and Marion are the grandparents I didn't have, coming over every few months and, when Jeanette was away for two weeks, filling in as babysitters. My girls love L's mum and idolize L's sister's daughters, in that way only two-year-old girls can of nine- and twelve-year-old girls. "You know," said L's mother to me during Passover dinner this year, "your girls are going to turn to you one day and say, what do you mean we're not Jewish?"

And then there is this. A few months after I moved to Manhattan from Brooklyn, the family next door moved out and a single woman moved in, so that with one exception, every apartment on my floor is occupied by single women. This is a lovely thing for us, not only to have neighbors who shower the girls with attention and care but because of what it does to the shape of our world. "Don't you wish you had someone to drink wine and watch TV with after the kids have gone to bed?" said a (married) friend recently and I felt myself prickle with the old defensiveness. Then I thought about it some more. So much of the fear I had about having children alone was a case of comparison-induced anxiety, just as having kids at forty-two was a very big deal to my mother and is not such a big deal today. When I collapse alone on the sofa at the end of the day, I'm at ease. Living where we do, it feels as if the girls and I are one expression of a majority trend, rather than an example of a failure to get married. Psychologically, this makes a big difference.

And then, shortly after the girls turned one, Oliver's girlfriend Heather got pregnant, the kind of gift I could have hardly dared hope for. Now he and I are on the phone to each other even more than we were before, two people raising babies far from the place they call home. "I'm going to offer you advice on your two-year-olds based on social psychology research and no practical experience whatsoever," says Oliver, "and you are going to offer me advice, based on zero experience, of what a newborn does to a conventional relationship."

Occasionally, I worry the girls don't see enough men. In a single week recently, one or the other of them identified Ariel Sharon, the late Israeli prime minister whose photo she saw in a newspaper, the bus driver who hangs out on the corner of our street between shifts, and Jim Broadbent as he appears on the cover of the movie tie-in book of Blake

Morrison's *And When Did You Last See Your Father?* as my dad, shouting out "Grandad!" at each of them and clapping with glee.

"I think all white men look alike to them," I grumbled to my dad on the phone, and that was before they yelled "Oliver!" at a Pakistani man in the street.

"I don't look anything like Ariel Sharon," said my dad, sounding wounded.

I also worry I'm spread too thin. When Oliver's baby was a week old, I visited him and Heather and felt fleetingly smug. The energy that two parents put into arriving at a mutual decision—does he need changing? Is he hungry? Should we take his temperature? What do you think? No, what do *you* think?—is catnip for single parents. Then, a few Sundays ago, the girls and I went to Brooklyn to have lunch with them all, and after the table was cleared, I watched as Heather handed the baby over to Oliver and went off to the gym. Just like that. An hour off. On the weekend. With a six-month-old at home. It was the most amazing thing I've ever seen.

One day, I receive an e-mail from a friend at the hospital, telling me he is sorry but he has some sad news. Dr. Y became ill shortly after the girls were born and he thought I'd want to know he had died. To my surprise, I start sobbing at my desk. I call L, who is sympathetic but baffled and then I call Oliver.

"I don't know why I'm so upset," I say. "But he was there on the most important day of my life. He brought them safely into the world."

"Well," says Oliver gently, "I would think that's enough." In all our years of friendship, he has never heard me cry like this. "It's good," he says. "You should do it more often."

It's true, I am softer now. I am grateful for absolutely everything. If the girls see a cat in the street and it makes them both laugh, I am happier than my happiest day before they were born. I find their arts and crafts unaccountably moving—although in duplication, they threaten to overwhelm us. The other day, when Dee Dee greeted her sister with the salutation "Hello, poop," I thought it was as funny as she did. And while I haven't sent Christmas cards featuring a photo of the three of us, it's only because I'm too lazy to send Christmas cards at all.

And yet I am still fundamentally me. When I have a bad writing day, it can't be salvaged by having a nice time with the kids. A good writing day, on the other hand, can make a rough time with them better. Sometimes, I think, if the girls hadn't happened, my life would have been void, and at other times, is this all it is? Not them. They are everything. But on the rare occasions I can separate the general "it" of motherhood from the specifics of mothering them, I can see the outline of how things might have been. Had it been possible to know how it was without actually doing it, I think I would have been fine. The thing I couldn't stand was not knowing.

What do I tell the children? On the train to Baltimore recently, I gave this more thought. I didn't travel much in the first year—a work trip to L.A. and another to Denver, both times Jeannette staying overnight with the girls—and the work trip to Baltimore is the first time in ages I've had a few hours to myself. I look out of the window as the New York suburbs bleed into the approach to Philadelphia and then the surprisingly rural scenery just outside Baltimore. After the failure of the first Facebook group, I had joined another, Single Twin Moms of Manhattan, made up of forty-seven members who, if I had to characterize them, I would say are not women crippled by low self-esteem. Most of us are too knackered to meet up, but it is a useful resource, discussing how to preempt Father's Day celebrations at preschool, or deal with two children and one pair of hands, or save money because, although many of us enjoyed a good lifestyle before the advent of twins, most of us are now chronically broke.

Some of the mothers on the site have shared experiences of using the donor exchange network first to identify, and then to meet up with, their twins' half-siblings through the donor. I admire the boldness of this, but I can't imagine doing it myself; the connection feels empty to me. On the other hand, my children may feel differently. They are lucky enough to be mirrored in each other, but the lure of a DNA connection that promises to fill in missing parts is probably much stronger than I think. I won't object if, one day, they want to go in search of their "half siblings", just as, if they want to find the donor when they're eighteen, that's fine with me, too. As they get older, the amount of space he takes up, so huge at the beginning, gets smaller and smaller, crowded out by the fullness of life, and as the train speeds along I realize I am looking forward to their asking the questions. I am excited to get it right and I am excited for them. They will have to think about identity earlier and in more sophisticated ways than some of their peers, and while I will tell them it's OK to be sad they don't have a dad, I will also point out that everyone has something about them that is different from others. As parents do, I find I am making a case for their exceptionalism. I chose this life, for them and for me, and there is power in that, too.

I knew I'd love them, of course. That was the whole point, to experience that love. What I had overlooked, along with so many other things, is that they would love me back. When my mother died, I thought no one would ever be as pleased to see me walk through a door again. Now, when I see the girls at the end of the day, they are so overwhelmed they can hardly cross the floor fast enough. Sometimes, Dee Dee simply drops to her knees and wails, "MUMMY." It's insane that this happens on a daily basis, the violence of it and what it does to my heart. Every time I see them I think, of course, you two; all my life I'd been wondering when you'd come along. I look at their faces and I'm at home in the world.

It is still hard. Someone always has a cold or is going through another sleep regression. There is never enough time, money or kitchen towel. Even two years in, the last diaper change before we leave the apartment—usually the third or fourth of the morning, which typically comes to light only once the girls are buckled into the stroller—nearly breaks me every time.

But it is summer again and we go to the beach as we did last year, loading up L's car and unloading it while the children fly out over the sand. They don't call themselves siblings but they fight as siblings and she and I yell at them indiscriminately when they do. "They're hers and he's mine," says L when anyone asks, which is the truth on which other truths lie. It is a long hot day and on the way home we sing "I've Been Working on the Railroad," and "Twinkle, Twinkle, Little Star," and a song L made up years ago for her nieces and which is still going strong, a tuneless number called "Sideways Seagull" that makes everyone howl when she sings it. When we get back to New York, we all go up to L's and while she makes dinner I give everyone a bath. Then we say good night and come downstairs.

It takes us a moment to settle. "Mummy, squash me," says Jane, as she says every night, and I lean back into the sofa to squash her. Then for ten minutes, they both shout, "Mummy, squash me, Mummy, squash me," and after I've squashed them we settle into the cushions to read. My dad and Marion bought the girls a collection of classic fairy tales and we read "Jack and the Beanstalk" and "Little Red Riding Hood," and then I start reading "Rapunzel." I find myself hesitating at the part where the princess is rescued by the prince, but the girls cry, "Mummy, read it!" and I do. They will understand it's one story among many.

There is a thud from upstairs as L gets her son ready for bed and I tell the girls to choose one more book. Shortly, we will go to the bathroom, and while one of my daughters stands on the toilet, I will hold the other while cleaning their teeth. Then I'll put them in their cribs, and after they've called for water, or milk, or whatever else they can think of to try to lure me back in, they will give up and go to sleep. For now things are quiet. Tomorrow is Sunday; I'm in no particular hurry. The girls lean into me, one on either side, and we read one last book and one more after that.

Acknowledgments

Thanks to Ann Godoff, Zoe Pagnamenta, Merope Mills, Oliver Burke-man, Heather Chaplin, Sarah Larson, Kate Fawcett, Tiffany Bakker, Janice Turner, Jat Gill, Niall Stanage, John Brockes, Marion Smith and those friends and family whose names have been changed, all of whom render absurd the notion of having a baby (and writing a book) "alone."

It is safe to say that without Judith Casimir or Annette Bougouneau not a single word of this book could have been written.

To those whose stories intersect most closely with my own: love and gratitude to fill one hundred more volumes. I promise I won't actually write them.